A Guide to
Living with
Hypermobility
Syndrome

of related interest

Body Intelligence
Creating a New Environment
2nd Edition
Ged Sumner
ISBN 978 1 84819 026 9

Curves, Twists and Bends
A Practical Guide to Pilates for Scoliosis
Annette Wellings and Alan Herdman
ISBN 978 1 84819 025 2

Managing Depression with Qigong
Frances Gaik
ISBN 978 1 84819 018 4

Meet Your Body
CORE Bodywork and Rolfing Tools to Release Bodymindcore Trauma
Noah Karrasch
Illustrated by Lovella Lindsey
ISBN 978 1 84819 016 0

Living with Dyspraxia
A Guide for Adults with Developmental Dyspraxia
Revised Edition
Mary Colley
Foreword by Victoria Biggs
Introduction by Amanda Kirby
ISBN 978 1 84310 452 0

A Guide to

Living with
Hypermobility
Syndrome

Bending without Breaking

Isobel Knight
Foreword by Dr Alan J. Hakim

SINGING
DRAGON

LONDON AND PHILADELPHIA

Figures 2.2 to 2.10 in Chapter 2 are kindly provided by Alex Stollery
Figure 2.11 on p.34 reprinted with kind permission from 'Ruby' from the Hypermobility Association Patient Forum
Figure 3.1 on p.51 and Box 3.2 on p.54 are reprinted with the kind permission of the Hypermobility Syndrome Association
Figure 10.1 photograph reproduced with kind permission from the dancer Mari Frogner and the photographer Alicia Clarke
All quotations from Professor Rodney Grahame are reproduced with his kind permission

First published in 2011
by Singing Dragon
an imprint of Jessica Kingsley Publishers
116 Pentonville Road
London N1 9JB, UK
and
400 Market Street, Suite 400
Philadelphia, PA 19106, USA

www.singingdragon.com

Copyright © Isobel Knight 2011
Foreword copyright © Dr Alan J. Hakim

Library of Congress Cataloging in Publication Data
Knight, Isobel, 1974-
 A guide to living with hypermobility syndrome : bending without breaking /
Isobel Knight ; foreword by Alan J. Hakim.
    p. cm.
 Includes bibliographical references and index.
 ISBN 978-1-84819-068-9 (alk. paper)
 1. Joints--Hypermobility. 2. Pain--Treatment. 3. Knight, Isobel, 1974---
Health. I. Title.
 RC933.K55 2011
 616.7'2--dc23
                              2011013057

British Library Cataloguing in Publication Data
A CIP catalogue record for this book is available from the British Library

ISBN 978 1 84819 068 9

Printed and bound in Great Britain

This book would not have existed without the support, vision and holistic insight of my truly wonderful physiotherapist, Katherine Watkins; so Katherine, this book is dedicated to you. Thank you from the bottom of my heart for everything you have done for me and for your help in what has been a very long (and unfinished) journey into transforming my body from being in such an unstable state to providing me with an improved quality of life. I feel that more is possible now than I could ever have imagined, and I know we haven't got there yet! My love and thanks, Isobel.

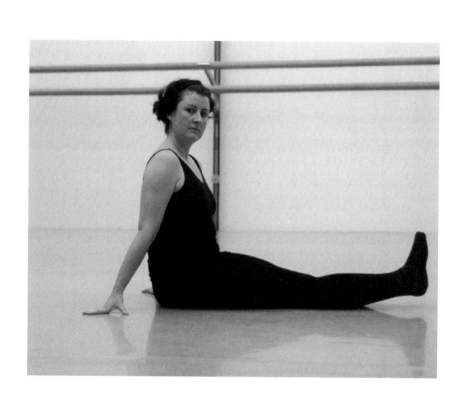

Contents

Foreword

Joint hypermobility syndrome is a complex beast. It is often so much more than being 'bendy' and in pain from multiple injuries, though coping with this can be difficult enough!

Since 2000, there has been an explosion of literature defining the problems associated with the syndrome. These can be physical or structural throughout the body, not just the joints. Also they can be disturbances of the nervous system, cardiovascular system, bowel or mood. The consequences are overwhelming, making it hardly surprising that living with the syndrome can seem daunting, isolating, frightening and depressing.

Support and advice for patients and clinicians continue to grow, and from a number of sources and points of view. That said, it can still take a very long time before the penny drops and someone recognises the diagnosis and points the individual in the right directions for help. Even then there can be reluctance among some (family members and medical personnel alike) to acknowledge the syndrome, the depth and breadth of its insult, and the psychosocial impact on an individual's wellbeing.

What Isobel Knight brings to the literature is something appealing and unique. Covering issues from childhood, adolescence and adulthood, she takes the reader through an autobiography, writing in a way that will be meaningful to so many living with and wanting to understand the syndrome.

Isobel hangs the breadth of the medical literature on her own experiences, the interventions of her therapists, and the shared stories of experts and of others with joint hypermobility syndrome. By incorporating interviews, blogs and poetry, including commentary from members of the Hypermobility Syndrome Association, Isobel weaves through every aspect of the syndrome.

The result is so much more than a synthesis of the medical literature in lay terms, and so much more than an individual's account of living with the syndrome. The variety of experiences and descriptions of the syndrome is rich and insightful.

This is a book for anyone who wants to understand the personal impact of joint hypermobility syndrome, as much as its clinical presentation and management, without all the medical jargon.

Dr Alan J. Hakim MA FRCP
Consultant Rheumatologist and Acute Physician
Director of Strategy and Business Improvement
Whipps Cross University Hospital NHS Trust, London
January 2011

Acknowledgements

There is an endless list of people who have made this book possible, including all the patients and dancers, teachers and medical professionals who have contributed in both time and interview and who have sent me such inspirational quotes. However, the following people deserve special thanks and acknowledgement.

Katherine Watkins, for being the first medical professional (in an extremely long line) who fully recognised all that was going on in my body and coped with the truly multisystemic nature of hypermobility syndrome. I think we have been required to rehabilitate nearly all my body systems, one way or another! Your patience, humour, support and generosity of time have been immeasurable. I hope that others will learn from your unique approach.

Professors Howard Bird and Rodney Grahame, for time in interview, and particularly to Howard, who generously saw me as a patient and diagnosed me initially, and for your time, expertise and help with editing the book, and ensuring what I said was correct! I am so lucky to have worked with the leading experts in HMS.

Teresa Kelsey, my ballet and Pilates teacher, who has helped me to strengthen and gain control of my hypermobility in a more safe and focused way – and has been supportive to me with her immense safe dance practice wisdom when I have been (often) managing injury and pain. Thank you also for your personal support and time in interview and discussion on the topic of hypermobility.

The Trinity Laban Pilates team have been extremely supportive and many hours have been spent in the Pilates studio under their watchful eyes – I am particularly grateful to Monica and Jessica, who have worked very closely with me.

Dr Emma Redding, Head of Dance Science at Trinity Laban, has been extremely supportive and I am so grateful for your time in reviewing the dance chapter. The MSc in Dance Science is a major part of what led me to write this book, and my learning outcomes of both the MSc course and my thesis opened the door into this fascinating topic. Trinity Laban is a truly unique establishment, and I wonder if the dynamic energy and creativity that exist there also facilitated my writing skills – I am sure that is true.

Donna Wicks from the Hypermobility Syndrome Association (HMSA) has been an inspirational and wonderful support who has kept me going during times of fatigue and writer's block. I would especially like to thank her for her help in reviewing Chapter 9 and for coordinating the support of the HMSA Medical Liaison Team on my behalf. I would also like to thank Natasha, Donna's daughter, for her unique contribution to Chapter 4.

I would like to thank Dr Jane Simmonds, who gave me time in interview and support in my writing endeavours. I would also like to thank Dr Alan Hakim for his time in reviewing my work.

My sincere thanks extend to Alex Stollery, who produced the beautiful illustrations in Chapter 2 – thank you.

Finally, I am extremely grateful to Jessica Kingsley Publishers for publishing this book and in particular to Lisa Clark and Victoria Peters for their time and patience in editing.

This book is dedicated to all those with connective tissue disorders – particularly those with hypermobility syndrome.

Introduction

Christmas is a time for seeing family and friends, eating lots of delicious food, maybe having some presents, and probably having a joyful and fun time. Maybe not. Aside from the fact that not everyone celebrates Christmas, it might not always be associated with being a 'happy' occasion, perhaps owing to family conflicts. Christmas might also be another of those occasions ruined by a painful and chronic medical condition that fails to take account of the good times. Christmas 2010 happened to be one of those for me.

I was fortunate enough to manage Christmas and Boxing Day relatively unscathed but by 27 December, when I was meant to be attending a big family lunch, my hypermobility syndrome (HMS) thought otherwise. I had severe neck spasm and pain in my lumbar spine. I was experiencing nausea, dizziness and a severe headache. I felt fatigued. My arms hurt. I disappointed my nearest and dearest, and had to go back home to London. The journey was a blur through my tears, which were not only self-pity but also the fact that yet again this condition had ruined another day where I was expected to put my body into a box and face a room full of people and act all jolly. There have been many times where I manage to do things when in pain, but there are different levels of pain and a range of other complicated symptoms attached to having joints with an excessive range of movement. Psychologically, the damage is deep and penetrating. I have experienced a lack of understanding from those apparently closest to me. I do not expect to be prescriptive in this book, but I do hope that this book will open the eyes (and hearts) of many people including the families and friends of those who suffer from HMS and also members of the medical profession who are not always as enlightened and aware of the difficulties related to this complicated medical condition.

If I could hope for one outcome of this book, it might be that the next person shows just a little more empathy and awareness of the plight of the person experiencing a chronic and challenging 'multisystemic' medical condition. Nobody can make the pain go away, and there are many other symptoms such as pain, fatigue, muscle stiffness, spasming, even things like dizziness and problems with bowels, all relating to the genetically inherited condition that is HMS. The syndrome has a symptomatic overlap with conditions like fibromyalgia and chronic fatigue and chronic pain syndromes, and is a connective tissue disorder caused by widespread faulty collagens. In a sense having a larger than normal range of movement and being able to produce interesting body postures (minus dislocations, which are also associated with hypermobility) are almost the least of the difficulties to be endured. It is tiresome and wearing explaining that despite the fact you might frequently look 'quite healthy' you often feel wiped out and in pain 'somewhere' in the body. The response of other people can make all the difference to coping with HMS.

CHAPTER 1

What is Hypermobility Syndrome?

WHAT IS JOINT HYPERMOBILITY?

Joint hypermobility can be described as having an excessive range of movement (ROM) in any given joint, above and beyond what would be considered the normal Gaussian range (Grahame 2003, 2009b; Nijs 2005; Simmonds and Keer 2007). An observed hypermobile joint might look inside out for example (see Figure 1.1) and a joint that is passively hyper-extended in excess of 10 degrees when measured with a goniometer (see Figure 1.2) would be considered hypermobile. It is certainly possible to have generalised hypermobility of joints and not have any difficulties or problems with the joints, and that is known as generalised joint hypermobility (GJH). It seems that most people have an awareness of their hypermobility, or 'being loose jointed'.

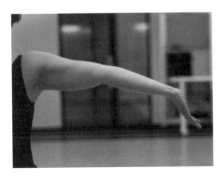

Figure 1.1: A hypermobile elbow joint

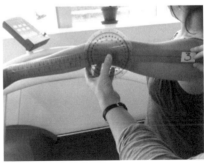

Figure 1.2: Measuring a hypermobile joint

HOW DID YOU KNOW YOU WERE HYPERMOBILE?

I don't know. I knew my joints were strange. I didn't hear the term academically until much later, but I always knew I had lax joints. I'd be told 'You sit weird' and you are 'a bit bendy' and that was how I ended up dancing. When I was growing up it was a bit like a party trick. Cousins asked me to do the splits and I could. (Zinzi Minot, contemporary dance student, Trinity Laban)

Last year I found out the name for being loose jointed, but hadn't thought about it before then, although I knew my elbows were hypermobile. Having hypermobile elbows is useful for finding things at the back of the sofa! (Mari Frogner, contemporary dance student, Trinity Laban)

DIFFERENCE BETWEEN GJH AND HAVING HMS

People sometimes question the differences between being generally hypermobile and having HMS. The main difference is that GJH is hypermobility which is normally asymptomatic, and not causing pain, whereas HMS is symptomatic and frequently causes pain (Grahame 2009a, 2009b; Grahame and Hakim 2008; Simpson 2006). There is a particularly high prevalence of hypermobility among gymnasts, acrobats, musicians and dancers, with up to 70 per cent particularly within the ballet and contemporary dance community, compared to 10–30 per cent within the non-dance population (Desfor 2003; McCormack *et al.* 2004; Ruemper 2008). Hypermobility could be described as a useful asset to dancers and performing artists because it often means that a person has improved flexibility and can achieve varied and interesting body postures (Simmonds and Keer 2007). Research has shown that GJH is desirable in the dance community, whereas having HMS is likely to be detrimental (McCormack *et al.* 2004; Ruemper 2008). The prevalence of hypermobility in the dance is so strong that a whole chapter has been devoted to the needs of hypermobile dancers (see Chapter 10). This book is primarily concerned with individuals with symptomatic HMS.

GENDER, AGE, RACE AND HMS

Generalised joint hypermobility has been identified as a gender-dominant condition and is more predominant in females and more common in African and Asian populations. When you look for HMS rheumatology clinics, the matrix of gender, race and type of presentation of HMS is complex (Grahame and Hakim 2006). If HMS is not influenced by other potential racial traits, for example usage of medical services and physical and emotional response to pain, and GJH is a baseline common finding in all, the population distribution of HMS patients in the UK would be expected to reflect the population distribution of GJH.

It is also known that hypermobility, in terms of flexibility, declines with age, hence it is sometimes necessary to ask adult patients to reflect on their youth, because if they could achieve challenging body postures (see Figure 1.3) or exhibit what might be defined as being double-jointed in the past, they might still have HMS (Bird 2005; Raff and Byers 1996). However, it seems that the symptoms of HMS do not decline with age.

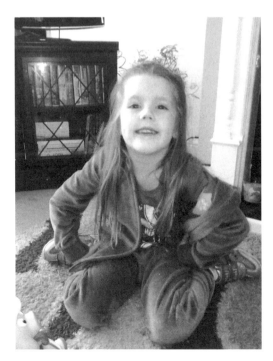

Figure 1.3: Hypermobile pose – sitting in the 'W' posture

WHAT IS A 'SYNDROME'?

A 'syndrome' is an association of several clinically recognised signs and symptoms reported by a patient that relate to one phenomenon. Well-known examples are irritable bowel syndrome (IBS), Asperger syndrome and chronic fatigue syndrome. For some medical conditions, the name or label of the condition can be crucial in order that the patient receives appropriate recognition of the difficulties that they might be experiencing, particularly where the patient looks deceptively well, frequently with an enhanced ROM, and yet is perhaps experiencing much pain and suffering (Grahame 2003, 2009a, 2009b). For such patients, the term syndrome should be applied adequately and accurately to reflect their symptoms.

In the 1990s a survey of UK rheumatologists identified the number of HMS cases being diagnosed as a proportion of all the patients seen in clinics. Given that the prevalence of HMS is not known, it is difficult to know how many cases were being missed or, more likely, diagnosed as fibromyalgia, chronic pain or chronic fatigue. A study of a city general rheumatology clinic suggested that up to half of cases with mechanical complaints (rather than inflammatory conditions like rheumatoid arthritis) had HMS (Grahame and Hakim 2006). If you extrapolate this information back to the UK survey in the 1990s, it suggests that then there was a big gap between the number of people presenting to clinics and the number given the diagnosis. Many people with HMS continue to struggle, in some cases for years, without a diagnosis despite multiple encounters with health professionals. Many are under-diagnosed perhaps because of their deceptive appearance of good health, or the medical professionals are not alerted to the syndrome and its many possible symptoms (Grahame 2009a, 2009b). In order to understand why the notion of a syndrome is so politically important in relation to this condition, it is relevant to understand the history behind the phenomenon of HMS.

The term 'hypermobility syndrome' was first coined by Kirk, Ansell and Bywaters in 1967, in response to the occurrence of musculoskeletal symptoms in otherwise 'healthy' individuals (Grahame 2003, p.4). Later on some experts wanted to refer to it as the 'benign joint hypermobility syndrome'. The term 'benign' has now been removed when associated with HMS because many people were angered that the prefix 'benign' did not adequately reflect the pain and many symptoms connected with the condition. Throughout the book, and for consistency, I will refer to it as hypermobility syndrome or HMS, although the syndrome is also known as joint hypermobility syndrome (JHS).

GENETICS AND CONNECTIVE TISSUE

HMS is a genetically inherited connective tissue disorder that is related to but distinct from two other connective tissue disorders – Ehlers-Danlos syndrome (EDS) and Marfan syndrome (MFS) (Grahame 2003). There are many types of EDS, with some of the more serious forms of the condition relating to cardiac problems. MFS is particularly associated with extreme tallness, very long fingers and highly extensible or stretchy skin which relates to all three conditions. Some experts refer to HMS and EDS Type III as the same condition while others believe that the distinction between HMS and EDS Type III can be differentiated by the skin extensibility and bony shape and articulation. This remains an area of contentious debate among medical experts, but currently it seems that EDS Type III might synonymously be known as hypermobility syndrome. Table 1.1 explains the different types of EDS and this book will still use the term HMS even if there are associations with EDS Type III in other literature.

HMS is therefore related to other connective tissue conditions and an autosomal genetic inheritance means that the person affected has one normal gene and one mutated gene, and one parent will invariably have the condition. Consultants often observe this genetic phenomenon when they meet families with the condition and, anecdotally, one consultant told me that he can tell from a handshake as to whether someone is hypermobile or not!

Table 1.1: Types of EDS

Type	Clinical features	Inheritance	Basic defect
Classical (formerly EDS Types I and II gravis and mitis)	Major: skin hyperextensibility; widened thin scars; joint hypermobility Minor: smooth velvety skin; molluscoid pseudotumours; complications of loose joints; muscle hypotonia; easy bruising; manifestations of tissue extensibility (hernia, cervical insufficiency, etc.); positive family history	Autosomal dominant	Abnormality of the pro alpha 1 (V) or pro alpha 2 (V) chain of the type V collagen encoded by COL5A1 and COL5A2 genes (in some but not all families)
Hypermobility (formerly EDS Type III hypermobile)	Major: generalised joint hypermobility; skin hyperextensibility and smooth or velvety Minor: recurrent joint dislocations; chronic limb and joint pains; positive family history	Autosomal dominant	Unknown
Vascular (formerly EDS Type IV arterial or ecchymotic)	Major: arterial/intestinal/uterine fragility or rupture; easy bruising; characteristic facial appearance Minor: hypermobility of small joints; tendon and muscle rupture; club feet; varicose veins; positive family history; sudden death in close relative	Autosomal dominant	Structural defects in the proα 1 (III) chain of collagen type III, encoded by the COL3A1 gene
Kyphoscoliosis (formerly EDS Type VI ocular or scoliosis)	Major: generalised joint laxity; severe muscle hypotonia in infancy; scoliosis present at birth and progressive; fragility of the sclera of the eye Minor: tissue fragility; easy bruising; arterial rupture; Marfanoid body shape; microcornea; skeletal osteopenia on X-ray; positive family history of affected siblings	Autosomal recessive	Deficiency of lysyl hydroxylase, a collagen modifying enzyme

Arthrochalasia (formerly included in EDS Type VII)	Major: severe generalised joint hypermobility with dislocations; congenital bilateral hip dislocation Minor: skin hyperextensibility; tissue fragility and scarring: easy bruising; muscle hypotonia; kyphoscoliosis; skeletal osteopenia on X-ray; positive family history	Autosomal dominant	Deficiencies of the proa (I) or proa 2 (I) chains of collagen type due to skipping of exon 6 in the COL1A1 or COL1A2 gene
Dermatospraxis (formerly included in EDS Type VII)	Major: severe skin fragility; sagging, redundant skin Minor: soft, doughy skin texture, easy bruising; premature rupture of foetal membranes; hernias	Autosomal dominant	Deficiency of procollagen 1 N-terminal peptidase in collagen

Source: Ehlers-Danlos Support Group 1997

Professor Howard Bird, consultant rheumatologist and HMS expert, said the following in an interview:

Autosomal dominant inheritance means that genes are carried on conventional rather than sex chromosomes so there is a 50 per cent chance the child will get it. Recessive inheritance is where it is overruled by other genes and that there is a one in four chance of an individual getting it. Autosomal dominant is the more common. All of that assumes hypermobility is a single inherited condition, but it is not. It is a common end point resulting from collagen inheritance though there is a stretching influence on collagen and from the articulated bony surfaces that can be inherited. Then there is the neurological aspect. People ask about their children. The probability of them having HMS is normally 50 per cent or less if one partner is not HMS and then the gene can 'be bred out' and can become less severe. If one partner is hypermobile and sometimes has a different type of hypermobility to the other partner, then it can get interesting and illustrate a double whammy effect with separate inherited material from each partner. (Professor Howard Bird, personal communication, 30 April 2010)

HMS, EDS and MFS are connective tissue disorders that relate to having faulty collagens resulting in excessive tissue laxity:

> Collagen is a major structural protein, forming molecular cables that strengthen the tendons, the skin and internal organs. Collagen provides structure to our bodies, protecting and supporting the softer tissues and connecting them with the skeleton. (Goodsell 2000)

Skin cream companies often advertise collagen as an essential ingredient so that we will retain our youth with soft but elastic skin. However, in people with HMS it is thought that the collagens are faulty and excessively elastic, hence the laxity of tissues throughout the body including skin, gut, lungs and joints (Bird 2007b; Grahame 2003). Once we begin to understand the ubiquitous nature of collagen (it occurs everywhere in the body) it becomes apparent that hypermobility is not simply about joints with an extra range of movement, but that it affects the body systemically. HMS is a 'multisystemic disorder' (Grahame 2009a, p.4).

TYPES OF HYPERMOBILITY

There are three different types of hypermobility, namely bony hypermobility, collagen-related hypermobility and neuropathic hypermobility. However, any one person will have varying combinations of these types of hypermobility, but one type may predominate (Bird 2007b). These classifications can be used to explain to a patient in more detail the predominant causes of their hypermobility, but other consultants might do things differently.

Characteristics of bony hypermobility

- Shallow joint sockets that might dislocate easily.
- Dancers and performing artists are easily able to do the box splits.
- Involves the joint articulating surfaces.
- Less hypermobility overall, but profound at a smaller range of joints.

Characteristics of collagen-related hypermobility

- In dancers and performing artists, the clues lie in the length of the preparatory warm-up and how long the collagens remain lax.

- Stretchy skin.

- More likely to have problems with other collagen structures, for example lungs (asthma), IBS (bowels) and weak bladder.

- More likely to be hormonally dominant, such as being affected by progesterone during menstruation in females.

Characteristics of neuropathic hypermobility

- Sometimes linked to a proprioceptive defect and new research is even highlighting problems with the reflex arc (Ferrell and Ferrell 2010).

- The clues to neuropathic hypermobility are the late walkers, clumsy gait and difficulties in retaining core stability.

- If linked to bony hypermobility, it is possible that some of the bones of the spine may be abnormal.

The overall management of HMS might depend to an extent on the prevailing 'type' or clinical classification of HMS (Bird 2007b). The management of HMS will be explored in detail in later chapters of the book, but it is useful to have an awareness of these types of HMS. The overarching treatment plan for HMS almost always relates to improving strength and stability and in order to protect the joints and their wide range of movement. However, for now this is a very crude explanation.

CONCLUSION

This chapter discussed the following points:

- HMS is a symptomatic variant of hypermobility that causes pain.

- GJH is asymptomatic hypermobility (Grahame and Hakim 2008; Simpson 2006).

- Many people with HMS struggle, in some cases for years, without a diagnosis despite multiple encounters with health professionals, therefore the prevalence of HMS is not known.

- HMS is a genetically inherited condition (Grahame 2003).

- HMS is a connective tissue disorder, with some physicians suggesting that HMS and EDS Type III are the same condition, and others advocating that it can be differentiated in the skin extensibility of EDS patients. The overall conclusion is that it is rapidly being accepted as EDS Type III (hypermobility type).

- HMS relates to faulty collagen proteins that affect the body systemically.

- GJH is prevalent in the performing arts community because being particularly flexible is a natural asset in the performing arts.

- HMS is prevalent in women and within the African and Asian populations.

- Some types of hypermobility decline naturally with age.

CHAPTER 2

Symptoms of HMS

In Chapter 1 the collagens in a person with HMS were described as faulty and excessively elastic (Bird 2007b; Grahame 2003). Collagen is systemic and it therefore becomes apparent that HMS is not simply about joints with an extra range of movement, but that it affects the body systemically. HMS is a 'multisystemic disorder' and its symptoms are holistic and far-reaching.

> People can be very healthy and active and then this domino effect occurs – I saw one in hospital today who is now very ill. The triggering is interesting. 'Multisystemic nature' – the joints can be the least major problem if you like, because if the internal organs and systems are affected then it is serious or incapacitating. I have seen since we have become interested in gut problems people who are much iller than I used to see. The medical profession has not caught on to this yet and people are misdiagnosed, misbelieved as it is not on the radar of doctors to think of hypermobility and systemic disease, so patients are said to be imagining the pain when it is not the case, it is not fair or true. (Professor Rodney Grahame, personal communication, 20 October 2010)

MAIN AND OVERARCHING SYMPTOMS

- Pain (widespread and localised).
- Fatigue.
- Joint pain.

- Regular soft-tissue trauma.

- Dislocations and subluxations.

- Slow healing.

- Overuse injuries.

Symptoms are further compartmentalised into the different body systems. The list in this book is not exhaustive, but is as accurate as both patient and academic-led research allows. Some symptoms overlap with other medical conditions. For example, asthma and IBS seem to have links with HMS and research has shown links with anxiety and HMS (Bird 2007b; Martin-Santos *et al.* 1998). Related conditions such as asthma and IBS are discussed in Chapter 7. This chapter explores in detail 'the why' behind the overarching symptom list.

SYMPTOMS RELATING TO THE SKIN

- Fragile skin and extensibility (see Figure 2.1).

- Easy bruising.

- Poor tissue healing and scar formation.

- Stretch marks.

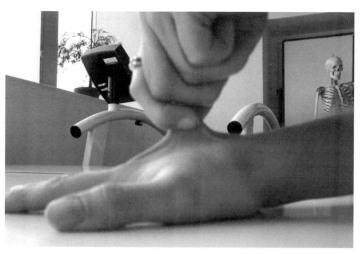

Figure 2.1: Skin extensibility with Ehlers-Danlos Type III (hypermobility type)

SYMPTOMS RELATING TO THE SKELETAL SYSTEM

- Dislocations.

- Subluxations (partial dislocations).

- Clicky joints.

- Hip dysplasia.

- Osteoporosis.

- Increased risk of fractures due to regular trauma.

- Increased risk of disc trauma due to excessive hinging at certain points in the spine.

- Increased risk of arthritis due to the potential of excessive joint wear and tear (joints taken beyond their normal ROM).

- Growing pains.

- Pubis symphysis disorder.

- Flat feet/fallen arches.

Figure 2.2 illustrates part of the skeletal system.

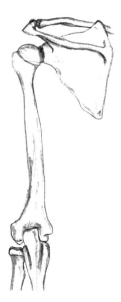

Figure 2.2: The skeletal system
Image by Alex Stollery

27

SYMPTOMS RELATING TO THE MUSCULAR SYSTEM

- Muscle tears.

- Increased risk of sprains.

- Increased risk of strained ligaments due to excessive joint ROM.

- Bursitis.

- Plantar fasciitis.

- Tendonitis.

- Muscle fatigue.

- Cramp.

- Muscle spasms.

- Muscle tics (twitches).

- Restless legs.

- Flat feet.

Figure 2.3 illustrates part of the muscular system.

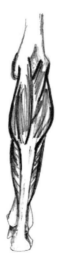

Figure 2.3: The muscular system
Image by Alex Stollery

SYMPTOMS RELATING TO THE NERVOUS SYSTEM

- Difficulties with proprioception.

- Pain related to fibromyalgia.

- Headaches.

- Impaired sensations in the body.

- Over-sensitivity.

- Restless legs.

- Clumsiness.

- Coordination difficulties.

- Poor reflexes.

- Numbness.

Figure 2.4 illustrates part of the nervous system.

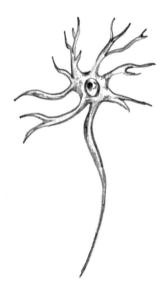

Figure 2.4: The nervous system
Image by Alex Stollery

SYMPTOMS RELATING TO THE CIRCULATORY SYSTEM

Postural orthostatic tachycardia syndrome (POTS) includes the following:

- Dizziness.

- Light-headedness.

- Fast heart rate (tachycardia).

- Headaches.

- Mental clouding.

- Varicose veins.

- Reynaud's syndrome.

- Changes in temperature.

Figure 2.5 illustrates part of the circulatory system.

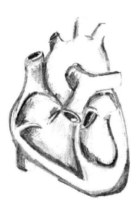

Figure 2.5: The circulatory system
Image by Alex Stollery

SYMPTOMS RELATING TO THE RESPIRATORY SYSTEM

- Difficulties swallowing.

- Asthma.

Figure 2.6 illustrates part of the respiratory system.

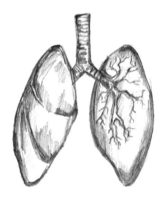

Figure 2.6: The respiratory system
Image by Alex Stollery

SYMPTOMS RELATING TO THE DIGESTIVE SYSTEM

- Difficulties swallowing.

- Indigestion.

- Nausea.

- Heartburn.

- Bloatedness.

- Constipation.

- Anal prolapse.

- Symptoms generally relating to IBS.

Figure 2.7 illustrates part of the digestive system.

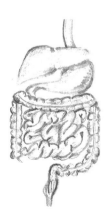

Figure 2.7: The digestive system
Image by Alex Stollery

SYMPTOMS RELATING TO THE URINARY SYSTEM

- Weakened bladder sphincter.
- Increased need for urination.

Figure 2.8 illustrates part of the urinary system.

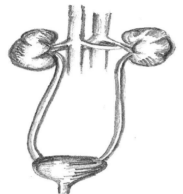

Figure 2.8: The urinary system
Image by Alex Stollery

SYMPTOMS RELATING TO THE REPRODUCTIVE (AND ENDOCRINE) SYSTEM

- Vaginal/uterine prolapse.
- Menstrual pain.
- Potential difficulties with pregnancy and childbirth.
- Increased likelihood of endometriosis.

Figure 2.9 illustrates part of the reproductive system.

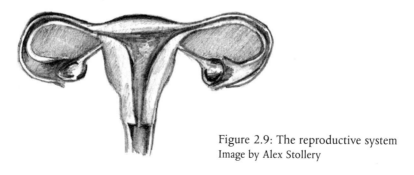

Figure 2.9: The reproductive system
Image by Alex Stollery

In the endocrine system, symptoms include increased joint laxity owing to progesterone in women during the menstrual cycle.

PSYCHOLOGICAL SYMPTOMS

- Anxiety.

- Depression.

- Memory loss.

- Difficulty concentrating.

- Poor sleep quality.

- Increased risk of self-harm.

- Learning difficulties.

Figure 2.10 illustrates part of the brain.

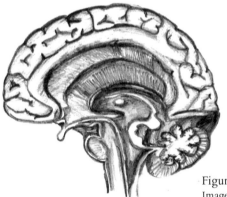

Figure 2.10: The mind and brain
Image by Alex Stollery

It is important to show the diverse range of symptoms that some HMS patients experience, which links to the faulty collagen genes and that the implications of having HMS are more complicated than having lax joints. Some people with HMS might have only a few of the listed symptoms, while others may suffer from a wider range of symptoms. For people who do have HMS, it is important that their symptoms are treated seriously and not ridiculed, and that the appropriate medical support is given to them, when and where necessary.

CHARACTERISTICS OF PEOPLE WITH HMS

Physiotherapists have observed their patients behaving in a variety of ways including 'fidgeting' and describe them as 'slouching [and] adopting end range of postures, such as entwining their legs' or habitually standing on one leg (see Figures 2.11 and 2.12) and 'resting on the lateral border of their feet in standing or sitting, producing a sustained stretch to the lateral ankle' (Keer 2003, p.79; Keer, Edwards-Fowler and Mansi 2003, p.96; Simmonds and Keer 2007, p.302). People with hypermobility are described as fussy, and 'frequently use their hands in an expressive way when talking' (Keer 2003, p.75). Children who may have HMS can even be labelled as inattentive or hyperactive because of fidgeting in class (Middleditch 2003). Such behaviours provide the physiotherapist with important clues to suspect the patient might have HMS, purely based on the way they move and behave (Keer 2003).

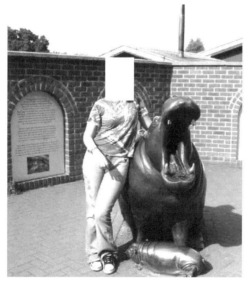

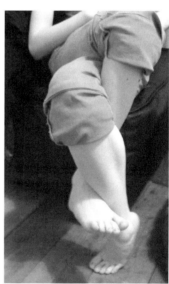

Figure 2.11: Patient with HMS showing an 'interesting posture'
Printed with kind permission from 'Ruby' from the Hypermobility Association Patient Forum

Figure 2.12: Legs 'entwined' pose

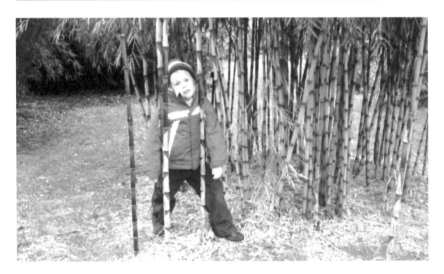

Figure 2.13: Ben, aged 7, requiring support!

But is it truly any wonder that patients 'behave' in this way with all these 'distractions' going on in their bodies, and the continuous instability that they experience owing to large joint ROM and the chaos of tissue laxity (see Figure 2.13)? My physiotherapist, Katherine Watkins, recognised my long medical and injury history and was able to suggest a diagnosis of HMS (later confirmed by a consultant rheumatologist): 'HMS is a global problem, and everything is so finely linked to other things...' (Katherine Watkins, personal communication, 22 April 2010).

So why do patients with HMS injure and experience some of the overarching symptoms listed on the previous pages?

PAIN

Acute pain is the result of regular trauma to bones and soft tissue. HMS patients are regularly injured, often through no fault of their own. The pain results from joints that are frequently working within an extra range of movement, therefore placing an additional strain on the surrounding soft tissue (Grahame 2003; Keer 2003).

The reasons why some hypermobile people have pain and others don't – that is a very difficult question to answer. There is no doubt that the most hypermobile people quite often have no pain, so there is no link between hypermobility and pain. Hypermobility can cause pain, but is not a direct relationship, and that the more hypermobile you are the more pain you get – we really do not know the answer to this question except, generally speaking, people who are fitter physically and take part in sport seem to be better protected than those who take less exercise, and within that group dancers are particularly well favoured because the nature of the work enables them to concentrate on precision and balance, particularly classical dancers, and gives extra protection. There are two populations of hypermobile people – those in hospital are the ones with problems. You'd think most people would have symptoms, but I suspect that, in the population at large, there is a much larger group who are hypermobile and do not have problems, never come near hospitals, so we don't see them. It is possible to be healthy, pain-free and hypermobile. We see the ones in hospitals who have problems. The number and variety of unrelated problems seems to increase, for example digestive problems and pain – we didn't know how important these were in the past. (Professor Rodney Grahame, personal communication, 20 October 2010)

DISLOCATIONS AND SUBLUXATIONS

Despite their increased range of movement, people with HMS report feeling stiff and experience clicking and popping sensations in their joints. They are prone to subluxations and dislocations (Simmonds and Keer 2007), which can make them feel vulnerable. Dislocations are a particularly challenging symptom. Dislocations and subluxations are caused by shallow bony sockets coupled with lax ligaments, resulting in the joint completely coming out of its socket as in a dislocation, or partially, as in a subluxation.

The following accounts are written by HMS individuals who experience dislocations and subluxations (HMSA online forum).

If I suffer an actual dislocation my first reaction is always shock. I remember just staring at the joint that is sticking out where it shouldn't be. However, the shock doesn't last long as my next instinct is to immediately put it back in. If it's my fingers I shake them which stretches the fingers out and allows the joints to pop back in. If it's my shoulder then I lie down on the edge of a bed then let my arm drop heavily downwards and it generally relocates the bone. If it's my foot, I generally fall to my knees in pain then sit down no matter where I am, take my shoe off and wriggle my foot manually until I feel my foot move freely again. Although I cry out in pain during the initial dislocation and there are often tears running down my face, I don't cry or sob – I'm too busy trying to stop the pain. I have always been able to relocate my joints myself; the thought of having to wait with my joint out of position is really scary to me.

If it's a subluxation, the pain can vary from almost dislocation pain to almost no pain whatsoever. After it happens I normally focus on making sure the joint is stable so that it's not going to happen again. Oh, and I swear like a trooper until the pain has eased. (Fiona)

My dislocations happen very quickly and always go straight back in again. Generally the pain is excruciating when it happens and will persist for several days afterwards. I can also feel the bones scraping against each other in the 'out' position and it's usually more painful as it goes back into joint again. I find I can't weight-bear properly afterward for at least a day or so (or grasp/reach if it's my shoulder or elbow).

I think everyone has a different experience of dislocations, even within their own bodies. The above description applies to my knees, hips and elbows but I can dislocate my shoulder painlessly, although I then get a huge amount of muscle and tendon pain a day or so after that can last for weeks. (Nemonie)

My hip subluxes (comes out of joint but slides back in easily) have been happening all my life and they don't always cause pain. When it comes out to the back and inside it gets stuck and I have a hard time getting it back in place for several days to a week. There is soft tissue damage and extreme pain. I can't walk or put weight on that leg and I have to use crutches till it goes back in. If it has been out long I usually develop bursitis and that can take a month or longer to heal. I need ice packs, heat packs, and pain medicine as it heals.

When I tore my shoulder joint the arm was hanging several inches lower than the other one. There was no way to get the shoulder back in place because it just came right out again. I had intense burning and searing pain that rolled over me in waves and made me sick to my stomach. I was in shock. My reaction was to grab the arm, hold it in place and to go to bed. I took codeine and thankfully it knocked me out. The next day it was still just as painful so I went to the Emergency Room. They did X rays and dispensed a sling and told me about the torn rotator cuff and told me to see an orthopaedic surgeon right away. I was given pain medicine, immobilization, ice, and after several weeks of rest I started physio. I ended up needing surgery to repair the shoulder but it tore again. For smaller joints I either put it back myself or just ignore it till it works its way back in place. ('Paw', 47-year-old female)

I don't seem to get the severe dislocation like many others, but I do have a rib that pops out. It is exceedingly painful and causes difficulty breathing, so have to breathe shallowly to reduce the pain. I've had my osteopath put it back before now, but it doesn't seem to be happening so often and only seems a bit out lately. It usually takes several days for the pain to go but it does subside slowly. (Dragondee)

SOFT-TISSUE TRAUMA

There are rarely signs of inflammation, but people with HMS often suffer from soft-tissue conditions, such as tendonitis and bursitis, plantar fasciitis, and carpal and tarsal tunnel syndromes (Grahame 2010; Simpson 2006). They undoubtedly suffer from more soft-tissue trauma owing to their tissue laxity and fragility of tissues. HMS is a genetic abnormality of the collagens which subsequently leads to biomechanical failure owing to the ligamentous laxity; factor in poor proprioception and it can be explained why there is an increased incidence of soft-tissue trauma in HMS patients.

SLOW HEALING

HMS individuals appear to take longer to heal. This might be owing to the properties of stretchy tissues. The skin is more fragile, it bruises more easily and scar tissue may not heal quite as well as in non-hypermobile people (Howse and McCormack 2009; Russek 1999). Soft tissues heal more slowly because the tissue structures are not well supported owing to the lax collagens and are simultaneously subject to further and continuous micro-tears and traumas. I know from my own experience that I have suffered continuous minor tears to my calf muscles simply because other aspects of my global muscular system, for example hamstrings and gluteals, were not functioning. This led to overuse in my calf muscles, frequent soft-tissue trauma and re-injury because the tissues never really healed properly.

OVERUSE INJURIES

Just had to stuff 1700 envelopes this weekend with bad arms and wrists! (D.W.)

People with HMS cannot tolerate overuse and the above quote is an example of an activity that is likely to cause a major flare up of pain in someone who already has problems with his or her arms and wrists. People with HMS do not tolerate overuse or repetition well, partly as a result of a lack of muscular endurance, which can lead to further injury (McCormack *et al.* 2004; Roussel *et al.* 2009). Hypermobile individuals might be less able to tolerate repetition because the muscles are working harder to control an extra range of movement, which might explain why their muscles fatigue sooner and they feel tired (Keer *et al.* 2003). HMS dancers and other people decondition and lose muscle tone quickly and often stop exercising because of injury or resultant pain. People with HMS may lose muscle tone quickly through time-loss from injury and because it is physiologically harder for them to strengthen their weaker collagenous tissues (Harding 2003; Simmonds 2003; Simmonds and Keer 2007). Muscle tissues atrophy greatly in the first five to seven days during inactivity, particularly the endurance slow-twitch muscle fibres. Muscles also atrophy in response to pain and fear, which might be a problem for some individuals with HMS (Keer 2003; Simmonds 2003).

The lumbar spine is one of the most mobile sections of the spine and in the hypermobile person often moves excessively: 'if this movement pattern is repeatedly reinforced through activities of daily living, it may lead to pain arising from overuse in the lumbar spine motion segments' (Simmonds and Keer 2007, p.303). Overuse then is exactly what it suggests it is – an area of the body working harder and doing more than it should at the expense of another area which is underutilised or not functioning correctly. My calf injuries were overuse injuries, and my lumbar spine pain was not only caused by hinging at the lumbar segments and a disc prolapse, but also because my lumbar and cervical spine were not biomechanically functioning optimally. Simply put, the muscular system is always having to work harder to control a larger ROM.

> When I stopped dancing I collapsed into my body. Then I started working in a pub, and pulling pints, and then had upper body problems which I hadn't had before. Problems before were in my lower back, hamstrings and gluteals. I was overusing one side of my body terribly and this was all new. I was very angry with my body for letting me down so much. Everyone can pull pints, all night, and I can't. I get pains everywhere. It is like painting a house – of course people get muscle ache, I do something like painting and I get in pain like you wouldn't believe. Just painting one wall – I get in a state and a half. My body is easily in pain. I cannot tolerate overuse at all – just working at the computer all weekend puts me in pain. I have to make sure I don't do the same things over again because I just get in pain immediately. (Mary, Pilates instructor)

FATIGUE

Fatigue is a significant problem for HMS patients: in a study of 170 adult women with HMS, 71 per cent reported that fatigue had a major impact on their lives (Bravo, Sanhueza and Hakim 2010). People with HMS are more likely to experience fatigue and flu-like symptoms (Simmonds and Keer 2007), because there is at least twice the amount of effort required constantly just 'to be' and that in itself is exhausting, so it might be understood to be a resultant problem from the continuous extra work the musculoskeletal system has to do in order to stabilise the body. The reasons underlying the fatigue in HMS are generally poorly recognised and understood.

Silent Support

More fatigued than a dead battery

My skeleton collapses against a wall for moral support

The wall acknowledges me silently as if it understands
about hard days.

(© Isobel Knight 2010c)

The muscles aren't equipped to deal with hypermobility without being re-educated. In order to do Pilates you need good functioning muscles. In untreated hypermobility all sorts of problems arise in the muscle system – in balance problems they all contribute to produce a locomotive system that is inefficient and not working well, so when you try for things requiring extra precision, it becomes very difficult. It takes re-education, and people who have never received that re-education just become not very efficient engines and the muscles aren't working properly. This is where fatigue links in and then you get muscle fatigue and a more general fatigue as the result of chronic pain. Sometimes the fatigue exceeds the pain, so I ask the patient which is most dominant, but both are major dampeners. (Professor Rodney Grahame, personal communication, 20 October 2010)

Sunday, 21 June 2009

Never ever let me dance under the influence of alcohol – ever again! I am paying the price today for doing some choreography which must have taken me into my most extreme hyperextensions systemically. Today I am paying for it, big time. I ache everywhere, and feel as though I have been run over by a bus. I even have pain in my fingers and hands. I would love to know what I managed last night because I can hardly move today. There is no doubt that HMS is a strange condition. Fatigue and pain are all part of it, but I can't sleep either because everything hurts too much! More baths and painkillers and perhaps some Bowen therapy or massage when I can get some! The only dancing I will be doing is horizontal dancing! (Isobel Knight)

PROPRIOCEPTION

Saturday, 7 March 2009

One of my ballet teachers this week noticed that my ankles are very hypermobile. This has not been pointed out before, as such. She noticed that my left ankle is at a peculiar and at a 'lethal' angle, medially when I am on the demi-pointe and is not in a straight line (bone stacked on bone) which it should be. She took immediate steps (no pun intended) in order to stop me doing pirouettes. She asked if I could feel that I was in the wrong place, which of course (being hypermobile) I could not. She had me looking at myself in the mirror in order to improve the alignment and asked me if I was doing foot strengthening exercises since she noticed my feet are much weaker in the centre, without the barre. I confirmed that I am.

One of the problems with people with HMS and EHS is that we lack proprioception – or an awareness of our joints in space and the end range of movements that our joints get into – this is partly why we get into the trouble that we do and are unaware of how 'bad' our alignment looks because we cannot sense it. (Isobel Knight)

Continual movement into an extra range of joint movement and joint instability, due to collagen laxity, can make people with HMS more prone to injury, because they have a poor sense of joint proprioception. Proprioception is determined by the spatial awareness of one's joints. For HMS individuals, their joint proprioception, particularly at the end range of movement into their hyperextension, can be impaired (Ferrell 2009; Hall *et al.* 1995).

> Is HMS a problem of the neurological system? My initial response is no. Because I see it as being a connective tissue disorder, affecting connective tissues that will indirectly affect the neurological system because there is collagen and connective surrounding some of the neurological pathways. But it is not a disorder of the neurological system. Proprioception might be poor because the tissues are lax. The sensory input isn't coming in, you are not getting the feedback from the joints or the tissues to the nervous system. It is not a disorder of the nerves to pick up, it is because they cannot sense the end range because they are not getting the feedback from the soft tissue. (Dr Jane Simmonds, personal communication, 14 August 2010)

A poor sense of proprioception could explain why people with HMS become injured, because of the lack of sensation in the joint at end of range (Batson 1992; McCormack *et al.* 2004; Nijs, Aerts and De Meirleir *et al.* 2006). People with HMS often have poor muscular tone and joint stability, increasing the likelihood of injury. Females have less muscle bulk and manage an increased ROM, which might explain why they suffer greater instability than males (Keer 2003; Ruemper 2008). There are more implications for women, whose symptoms can worsen prior to menstruation, caused by an increase in the hormone progesterone, which further relaxes collagen. In female adolescents, both growth spurts and the onset of menstruation can make symptoms such as pain and joint instability worse, increasing the overall risk of injury and further impairing proprioception (Bird 2004, 2007a; McCormack *et al.* 2004; Nijs *et al.* 2006).

Proprioception is about this ability to know where you are in space. In hypermobile people the proprioceptors are basically not giving the right feedback. It is very easy to understand this with the hypermobile knee and elbow and imagine this in the rest of the body as well. It is keeping the spaces open not just muscularly, but it is about re-learning where the body is in space. I think that for people in a lot of pain this is quite something because they are in a lot of pain partly because they are hanging into certain parts of their body because they can't feel they are doing it. The first thing we need to do is to make people aware of where they are in space, even when standing around. The proprioceptive system is so such a basic system in being human if it is not really working 100 per cent what is happening is, and I don't feel it so much myself because I have done so much body work, but for others this sense of not knowing where you are in space is basically eroding a sense of identity and not knowing who and where you are literally, which makes the condition so debilitating. (Mary, Pilates instructor)

The resultant difficulties of poor proprioception are all linked into the other difficulties with HMS such as overuse, a susceptibility to soft-tissue injuries and dislocations and subsequent poor healing due to constant reinjury. Figure 2.14 might aid the explanation. If one cannot sense where one's joints are, the probability of an incident or trauma is heightened (Ferrell and Ferrell 2010).

The reasons underlying why people with HMS have poor proprioception might link into the tissue laxity of the soft tissues. Motor development is frequently delayed, and also relates to impaired proprioception since motor coordination is dependent upon accurate proprioceptive feedback (Ferrell *et al.* 2004). If continuous injury is factored in, the body is continuously getting the 'wrong' motor information about where it should be. It seems that, in HMS individuals, there is a neurophysiological dysfunction, possibly relating to problems of the autonomic nervous system (ANS), which controls heart rate, temperature and bowel function (more in Chapter 7), which we know also causes such problems as dizziness (Ferrell and Ferrell 2010).

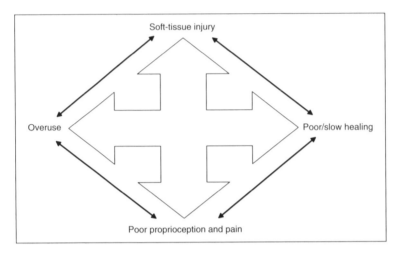

Figure 2.14: The close relationship between injury, pain and healing

Assessment for proprioception can be conducted for example using the Romberg balance test (see Figure 2.15), a rather crude test of balance (stork pose). It seems likely in the Romberg balance test that:

> In asymptomatic hypermobile subjects results are comparable to normomobile individuals, suggesting that hypermobility per se may not be the causative factor for the impaired balance in JHS patients, but rather that there is an associated neurophysiological dysfunction in HMS. (Ferrell and Ferrell 2010, p.101)

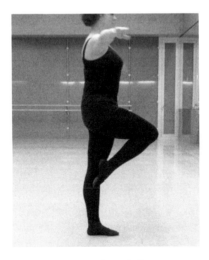

Figure 2.15: Romberg balance test, conducted with eyes shut

MANAGEMENT OF PROPRIOCEPTION

It is possible to improve proprioception through exercise. In one study 16 of the 18 subjects measured showed 'very significantly improved' performance on a balance or wobble board following hamstring and quadriceps exercise ($p<0.001$). Exercises also led to improved strength and reduction in pain and improved quality of life (Ferrell *et al.* 2004). This is highly significant, and why it is important for HMS patients to be gently and slowly rehabilitated with exercises, since improving muscle tone and reconditioning will also improve proprioception and potentially reduce the number of ongoing traumas. Clumsiness, balance and fitness should also improve (Ferrell 2009; Ferrell and Ferrell 2010).

The following can help in the management of proprioceptive dysfunction:

- Improving joint stability by means of joint stabilising exercises.

- Avoiding end-of-range joint positions which could be potentially damaging.

- Reversing muscle deconditioning which accompanies muscle disuse.

- Through appropriate aerobic exercise, enhance fitness and stamina.

- Improve core stability.

- Manage chronic pain by pacing and coping strategies.

- Improve proprioception by employing appropriate exercises.

(Ferrell and Ferrell 2010, p.101)

CONCLUSION

In this chapter we have looked at just how multisystemic HMS is and some of the overarching and resulting symptoms from having tissue laxity such as pain, frequent soft-tissue trauma, overuse, dislocations, fatigue and problems that result from having poor proprioception. All these resultant symptoms are related, and in rehabilitating them (most likely with medical support) they all have to be addressed in a multidisciplinary way (with different medical experts), over time. The underlying message about exercise is crucial and it has a highly significant factor in improving the management of HMS. It is the one thing that you can do for yourself as the patient, with appropriate support.

Pain management is discussed in Chapter 6. Information about other related HMS conditions is included in Chapter 7.

CHAPTER 3

Diagnosis of HMS

HMS is a condition where pain is a major problem, but the range of symptoms extends systemically and it is a far more complicated condition than simply having hypermobile joints. So how would you know whether you had HMS? Although a good family doctor or an experienced physiotherapist might be aware that you have HMS, the condition is ultimately diagnosed by a consultant rheumatologist.

Hospital consultants are becoming increasingly specialist, for example some orthopaedic (bone) consultants may specialise in only one area of the body – perhaps the knee joint. In a condition which is so systemic it is sometimes necessary to view the whole body and not just one tiny component, and this is where rheumatologists come into their own. Although they look at joints and joint inflammation, they will also want an overview of a patient's general health and prior medical history. Although other specialists will do this, if the rheumatologist does this, an accurate diagnosis of HMS can be made, ensuring holistic and ongoing patient care. Rheumatologists are good at looking at the body in a multisystemic way and will take care to look at whether a potential patient with HMS also has trouble with their digestive system. As seen in Chapter 2, HMS can affect the whole body, and not just one or two joints.

DIAGNOSING HMS

Before seeing a consultant rheumatologist it might be possible to identify personal hypermobility by answering the five diagnostic questions in Box 3.1, although this should not be a substitute for medical advice. This would be helpful for more mature patients since hypermobility declines with age and it is sometimes useful for mature patients to reflect upon their youth (Bird 2005; Raff and Byers 1996). As the criteria outcome predicts, a score of two or more out of five would suggest an 80–90 per cent chance of hypermobility (Hakim and Grahame 2004). If you have the appropriate score and other symptoms, it would be sensible for you to seek advice from a general practitioner (GP) with the possibility of a referral to a rheumatologist, if deemed beneficial. However, HMS is not always easy to diagnose (before seeing an expert).

BOX 3.1 FIVE DIAGNOSTIC QUESTIONS

Do you have hypermobility syndrome?

Here is a five-part questionnaire to identify hypermobility. If you answer yes to at least two of the five questions, there is an 80–90 per cent chance you are hypermobile.

1. Can you now (or could you ever) place your hands flat on the floor without bending your knees?

2. Can you now (or could you ever) bend your thumb back to touch your forearm?

3. As a child did you amuse your friends by contorting your body into strange shapes or could you do the splits?

4. As a child or teenager did your shoulder or knee cap dislocate on more than one occasion?

5. Do you consider yourself to be double-jointed?

Source: Professor Rodney Grahame and Dr Alan Hakim, Department of Rheumatology, University College Hospitals, London

Professor Rodney Grahame has been instrumental in improving awareness among rheumatologists about the plight that many HMS patients have to go through and the hope is that this figure will radically improve with doctors being made more aware of HMS and research providing an increasingly clearer picture of the range of symptoms connected to HMS.

THE BEIGHTON SCORE

The most frequently used method of diagnosing HMS is the Beighton score, which was devised in the 1970s to measure hypermobility in rural Africa, and to provide indications of the propensity of hypermobility in this population. In order to assess as many people as possible, the scoring system was devised to be a rapid assessment while clinically simple to measure.

The Beighton score involves a series of nine measures including measurements of spinal flexion, thumb adduction, little finger, and elbow and knee extensions. Historically, some experts have disagreed about the determinant score for a diagnosis, with some in particular suggesting that the cut-off criteria should be different for men and women, because women score higher (Russek 1999). It is now accepted that a score above four gives a diagnosis of generalised hypermobility (GH). The maximum score is nine and you would be considered hypermobile if you scored greater than four moves out of the nine: this is a 'major' criteria for hypermobility. This score reduces to three out of nine for those over 50 years old since hypermobility declines with age. Figure 3.1 gives an overview of the assessment movements required for the Beighton score, and Figures 3.2 to 3.6 show the individual measurements. Sometimes a measuring implement known as a 'goniometer' might be used in order to measure a joint range of movement, as seen in Figure 3.5.

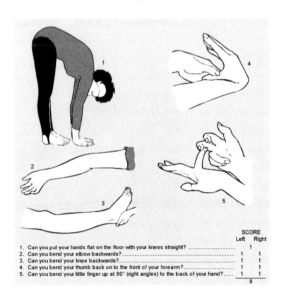

Figure 3.1: The Beighton score
Printed with kind permission from the Hypermobility Syndrome Association

51

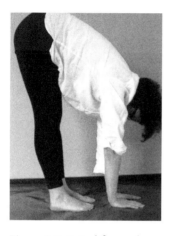

Figure 3.2: Spinal forward flexion

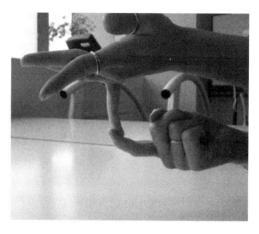

Figure 3.3: Little finger with angle at 90 degrees

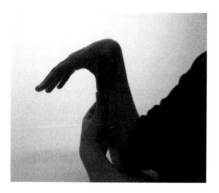

Figure 3.4: Thumb abduction (positive score)

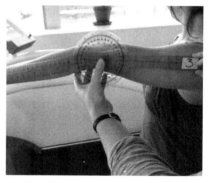

Figure 3.5: Measuring the elbow joint using a goniometer

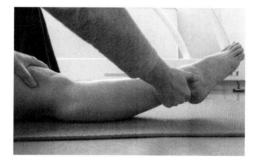

Figure 3.6: Assessing hypermobility of the knee

Historically, the diagnosis of hypermobility has not been without controversy, and remains a topic of contentious debate among clinicians. Hypermobility was originally diagnosed using the Carter Wilkinson scale, which included some of the movements listed in Figure 3.1. However, the assessment of forward flexion was absent, and instead excessive dorsiflexion and eversion of the foot were present. The Beighton score superseded the Carter Wilkinson scale, and is still considered the benchmark in the measure of hypermobility (Carter and Wilkinson 1964; Russek 1999). One problem with the Beighton score is that it assesses only a few joints. As previously discussed, its original use was for rapid assessment of joint hypermobility in rural Africa.

The Carter Wilkinson scale and the Beighton score have been used to compare musculoskeletal characteristics in HMS. Excessive ankle dorsiflexion and little finger dorsiflexion beyond 90 degrees were the two most common findings (Bulbena *et al.* 2004; Grahame 2003; Russek 1999). The Beighton score looks at only a small range of joints and cannot quantify hypermobility and joint laxity (Bird 2007b). Therefore, some rheumatology consultants opt to examine other major joints, such as the hips and shoulders, in order to provide a more comprehensive assessment of hypermobility across the body. The Barcelona scale includes a wider range of joints and one particular measure of hypermobility, the Contompasis score, also provides different grading for the moves it measures; so the greater ROM there is in a joint, the higher the points score. This might be one way of quantifying hypermobility.

The number of joints affected does not necessarily correlate with the amount of symptoms experienced in the affected individual. There is, therefore, a need for a further measure in assessing HMS, which is the underlying reason for the Brighton criteria (Grahame 2003, 2007, 2009a; Russek 1999).

THE BRIGHTON CRITERIA

While the Beighton score can determine generalised joint hypermobility, which is hypermobility that is asymptomatic and not causing pain, the diagnosis of HMS requires an additional set of criteria, namely the Brighton criteria, which were formalised by Grahame (2000) in order to capture the multisystemic nature of HMS (see Box 3.2).

BOX 3.2 BRIGHTON CRITERIA

Revised diagnostic criteria for HMS

Major criteria

- A Beighton score of 4/9 or greater (either currently or historically).
- Arthralgia for longer than three months in four or more joints.

Minor criteria

- A Beighton score of 1, 2 or 3/9 (0, 1, 2 or 3 if aged 50+).
- Arthralgia (over three months) in one to three joints or back pain (over three months), spondylosis, spondylolysis/ spondylolisthesis.
- Dislocation/subluxation in more than one joint, or in one joint on more than one occasion.
- Soft-tissue rheumatism with more than three lesions (e.g. epicondylitis, tenosynovitis, bursitis).
- Marfanoid habitus: tall, slim, span/height ratio >1.03, upper:lower segment ratio less than 0.89, arachnodactyly (positive Steinberg/wrist signs).
- Abnormal skin: striae, hyperextensibility, thin skin, papyraceous scarring.
- Eye signs: drooping eyelids or myopia or antimongoloid slant.
- Varicose veins or hernia or uterine/rectal prolapse.

HMS is diagnosed in the presence of two major criteria, or one major and two minor criteria, or four minor criteria. Two minor criteria will suffice where there is an unequivocally affected first-degree relative.

Source: The Hypermobility Syndrome Association, reproduced with written permission

The Brighton criteria are crucial to the diagnosis of HMS because it is a multisystemic condition and so there are questions in the Brighton criteria relating to joints, skin and blood vessels as all these can be affected in patients with HMS and are ultimately related to faulty collagen fibre structures, systemically (Russek 1999; Simpson 2006). In addition to widespread pain, there are a range of conditions that are linked to HMS because of the known tissue laxity and resultant faulty collagen fibres. Some examples are asthma (Bird 2007b; Simmonds 2003), varicose veins (Russek 1999), rectal or uterine prolapse (Simpson 2006) and autonomic dysfunction – symptoms of dizziness, palpitations and light-headedness (Grahame 2003). Furthermore, there is an overlap in diagnosis between HMS and two other connective tissue disorders, Marfan and Ehlers-Danlos syndromes; particularly in relation to assessment of stretchy and thin skin with EDS and overly long fingers and thumbs in Marfan syndrome (Bird 2007b; Grahame 2007; Raff and Byers 1996; Russek 1999; Simpson 2006). As the Brighton criteria are developed in future, features of HMS such as cardiovascular autonomic disturbances such as rise in pulse or drop in blood pressure on standing, and bowel symptoms similar to IBS, are likely to appear in the list of systemic things that doctors should look out for.

WHAT HAPPENS WHEN YOU SEE A CONSULTANT RHEUMATOLOGIST?

What follows is my own account.

The assessment was very thorough because Dr H needed to know my medical history, including information about other family members because of the genetic component to the condition, and he was able to confirm I have HMS. We concluded that I had probably inherited the 'shallow' hip and shoulder sockets from my maternal family, and the ligamentous laxity from my paternal family. Although H thought it was a general 50/50 split between the two aspects of hypermobility, we thought conclusively that the bony component might be slightly dominant.

H's assessment of my joints was very interesting. He didn't just do the standard Beighton score, but looked at a far greater range of joints than is assessed in the Beighton score. For example, H looked at my shoulders, hips and ankles and determined that my hips and shoulders are hypermobile and demonstrate greater mobility than other Caucasian women of my age, meaning it was not acquired hypermobility through dance.

H had been particularly interested in my reporting a significant difference in leg length and on examination of my spine suspected that I have what he calls an 'S-shaped twist' on one side of my spine. He also noticed that my shoulders were uneven, and that (as I knew) I hinged in a particular area of my lumbar spine. All this might explain my injury pattern and the compensations that are being made biomechanically in my legs, to account for this structural imbalance. In order to determine diagnosis H needs me to have a lumbar spine and pelvic X-ray. Following that he will be able to make further recommendations to my physiotherapist and the Pilates team about how this might be corrected. (Isobel Knight)

I remember my consultation very well because I recall being asked if I did any interesting or unusual 'party tricks' that are so common among hypermobiles – for example taking shoulders out of joint, showing off double-jointed thumbs, sitting in the 'W' posture (see Figure 1.3). I said that I did not, but then went on to shoulder my leg and then sit with my legs in the double-lotus position for the rest of the consultation, showing true hip hypermobility. It was interesting discussing the possible genetic links in my family, or where and how I had developed my hypermobility. In fact I was asked to bring to clinic my medical history and my consultant went through each point and linked it or not with me having HMS. He was very interestingly able to hypothesise that my shallow joint sockets were inherited from my maternal family, while the ligamentous laxity most probably came from my paternal family. I brought with me a long history of chronic pain and recurrent injury and a range of other symptoms I had always had. It was not until H pieced all this together that the diagnosis of HMS became complete and apparent and perhaps explained a myriad of problems.

When Dr H retired, I was sent to University College Hospital in London for future management. Only the more severe cases of HMS end up in hospital and there are many people with HMS who do not need hospital management, although they will undoubtedly need physiotherapy or Pilates to manage their joint laxity. HMS is a holistic condition and it increasingly requires rheumatologists to involve other medical experts in the care of HMS patients.

Tuesday, 5 October 2010

I was seen for a very thorough review by a leading rheumatologist in central London. These are the main summary points:

- Sleep/fibromyalgia – writing to GP to put me on Amitriptyline again starting at a low dose. Getting sleep sorted is crucial.

- Bladder – urodynamic assessment of my bladder to see what they find as this predates endometriosis, but is getting worse.

- Postural Orthostotic Hypotension (POTS) – referral to another doctor.

- Heart – referral for an echocardiogram given family history.

- Feet – referral to podiatrist – said I had slightly flat feet. Not something I was particularly aware of, but will see what they say.

- Neurologist – I am being referred re the 'things' going on in my spine. She said she had never seen that ever before. She said they weren't muscle spasms as such, but thought this should be investigated further as they have been going on for some time and have become worse over time.

(Isobel Knight)

Anna's story

Although I have experienced problems associated with joint hypermobility since birth, I was not diagnosed with HMS until the age of 37. The issue that finally led to an appointment with a rheumatologist was persistent pain in my left shoulder and unresolvable 'tennis elbow' as a result of carrying my second child on my hip when she was a baby. It was at the GP appointment that led to the referral that I described the various joint-related problems I had been experiencing over the last year and throughout my life.

Despite my life-long interaction with the health system, beginning at age 6 months with treatment for a shallow hip socket, followed by dislocating knees since age 4 necessitating surgical intervention as a teenager, culminating in spondilolysthesis diagnosed while undertaking a degree of nursing resulting in a spinal fusion (along with a few minor complaints thrown in, such as jaw problems, 'tennis elbow', painful wrists etc.), never before had a health care professional commented on the possibility of a link.

Her suggestion that a referral to a consultant rheumatologist was advisable felt at the same time reassuring and alarming. Awaiting the appointment, yet more problems arose: driving the car more than usual resulted in bursitis in my left ankle and inflammation in my right knee, as well as exacerbating the damage in the shoulder and elbow.

Before the appointment I made a note of all of the joint-related difficulties I had experienced. I wanted to be sure to mention everything. This was the first time that I had ever looked at the different problems 'on the same page'. It looked and felt rather overwhelming and I realised that I could not think or talk about my life without reference to my physical problems. Apart from being an intrinsic part of my experience of life, my physical difficulties had shaped my life to a great extent. At the appointment the consultant listened, asked some questions, made notes and examined me physically. She gave me an ARC booklet about joint hypermobility and HMS and said something along the lines of, 'I think you might find this helpful'. She skilfully administered a cortisone injection to my shoulder and we left the appointment, booked in to return in six weeks.

At the time I was confused: Why had she not made a 'formal diagnosis'? Did I have HMS or not? Perhaps she wasn't sure. With hindsight I feel that this approach was extremely helpful: Not directly 'telling' me that I had HMS allowed me to then find out about it at a pace that suited me emotionally. The more I read the clearer it became that I did indeed have HMS and that this was what had affected me throughout my life. Over the next year or so I saw the consultant several times as she referred me for shoulder surgery and for a physio programme aimed to strengthen various joints. One appointment particularly stays in mind, at which we talked about the need to manage the symptoms since the condition could not be 'cured'.

Attending a local NHS 'Expert Patient' course further helped me to come to terms with my reality. While it was reassuring to know that I was, on the whole, already on the right track with regard to managing the condition, the most significant aspect of the course for me was simply being there. The course was for people with long-term health issues. Me being there meant that I really did have a long-term health issue! I think that there is a difference between knowing something to be the case and really feeling or believing it to be so. It has taken me a couple of years to really assimilate this information into my reality. I remember at times not feeling very connected with the idea of having HMS and on the journey towards coming to terms with it, I have experienced different phases often dominated by one particular emotion: For a while I felt happy and relieved that an explanation had been found for the difficulties I had experienced. I then felt angry that it had taken so many years for the problem to be identified and furious that I had not had the information earlier on that may have prompted me to have made different choices in my life and thus incur fewer problems. Next I felt miserable at the prospect of having no escape from HMS and wondered how I would cope. Finally I started to feel more resolved to the idea of having a long-term health condition and more determined not to give in to despair.

Although difficulties old and new do persist (more recently I have suffered plantar fasciitis and pain higher up in my spine), I feel that I have been able to go a long way towards coming to terms with having HMS. I don't like it or want it but I do accept that I have to put up with it and live with it the best I can. (Anna, aged 37)

CONFIRMING THE DIAGNOSIS

Last week I had an appointment with Prof. Grahame. He diagnosed me with Ehlers-Danlos hypermobility type. He explained that because discs are made from collagen, mine have been unable to repair themselves once injured; and that they never functioned properly in the first place. This explains my disc degeneration and annular tears, and also why the facet joints have been under so much strain that I developed osteoarthritis at 27. He was so sympathetic and wonderful and he knew everything I was going to say before I had a chance to speak! He also mentioned that EDS causes pain signals to be amplified more than normal through the spinal cord. This means that a 'normal' person with my back problems wouldn't be in as much pain as I am. That explains why all the doctors I've seen treat me like I'm making a huge fuss over nothing! (Louisa, aged 27)

For me, finding out that I had HMS was quite a shock and I was initially upset about it. I knew I was generalised hypermobile from my teenage years when a ballet teacher had told me about my 'swayback knees' but I had no idea that my regular calf tears, my back pain, fatigue, poor sleep patterns, anxiety, depression, asthma, IBS, poor coordination, poor concentration and endometriosis might also be linked to having HMS. My physiotherapist was the first to suggest I had HMS and some months later this was officially confirmed by a consultant rheumatologist. When I had a diagnosis I could start to put together all the pieces of the jigsaw that for me made up HMS. Once I was able to accept this I was able to look at where I went from there, and although I am a great deal more 'stable' than I was, it has taken about four years to attain this level of control over my unstable body. I think I would add unstable mind as well because, now that my body feels stronger and more stable, I feel calmer in my mind and have much less difficulty with mood swings than I did in the past.

My journey into managing my HMS probably starts in 2006 when I was sent to attend a pain management course and this and pain management in general are discussed in Chapter 6. The rest of my recovery stemmed from regular physiotherapy and Pilates sessions and these are documented in later chapters. Additionally the Bowen technique, a gentle soft-tissue therapy, has been instrumental in helping with pain and management and some of the subsidiary symptoms of HMS such as fatigue and low energy levels. Feldenkrais, a form of movement therapy, has been extremely invaluable, and of course the acid test in all of this has been in my being able to restart and continue safely with classical ballet classes, something that prior to 2006 had been beyond my wildest dreams.

CHAPTER 4

Children and HMS

I hadn't realised how widely the syndrome could affect you. I already knew I had double-joints, but no one ever explained it to me. My gym teacher at school was a physiotherapist and could see that I wasn't coping with most gym things – vaulting and climbing bars – could see I wasn't strong enough and stopped me doing most of that including ball games because I was always spraining my ankles, so I couldn't do a cross-country run, or play hockey, which was absolute murder. I didn't know why I hated hockey so much, but then that was stopped and I was allowed to go riding, which I enjoyed. I haven't got hypermobile joints everywhere, but I have toes, ankles and hips and fingers and wrists, but not elbows and knees! (Grace, aged 65)

LATE WALKING

For many parents, the first time they realise that there might be a potential problem with their child is when they learn to walk late, or perhaps bottom shuffle rather than crawl (Knight and Bird 2010). This is a very common occurrence in the HMS population, with HMS babies in one study walking at an average of 15 months, with some being considerably later than the usual 12 months. Reasons for the bottom-shuffling behaviour as opposed to crawling particularly link to those children who have hypermobile elbows and the late walking relates to general instability and poor coordination (Adib *et al.* 2005; see also Maillard and Murray 2003). Children attending rheumatology clinics (and adults) are asked whether they bottom shuffled or were late walkers, because this does indicate hypermobility.

DEVELOPMENTAL COORDINATION DISORDER

If hypermobility is not recognised initially in young children, as they grow and develop there are other 'signs' that will indicate that their hypermobility is a hindrance for them. Clumsiness, fidgeting behaviour and poor balancing skills are very common in hypermobile children owing to their joint instability, just as is the case with adults (Maillard and Murray 2003). There are links with HMS and difficulties with motor coordination and learning and developmental coordination disorder (DCD; previously known as dyspraxia) (Adib et al. 2005; Jaffe et al. 2005; Kirby and Davies 2007). In a study involving 68 children with HMS (mean age 9.7 years) and 58 children with DCD (mean age 8 years), a questionnaire to parents revealed a huge overlap in the difficulties encountered with both groups in terms of problems with using scissors (66% HMS, 69% DCD), problems with writing (53% HMS, no stats for DCD) and ball skills (57% HMS, 70% DCD), difficulties with spelling (49% HMS, 55% DCD) and difficulties with making friends (41% HMS, 47% DCD) (Kirby, Davies and Bryant 2005, p.435).

> The reported difficulties with higher functions of the brain (e.g. spelling and calculation) and social interaction of the individual may be a primary symptom of central nervous system dysfunction and could also be a result of motor deficit and its subsequent impact on the ability of the child to interact with his/her environment. (Adib from 'Letters to editor', in Kirby et al. 2005, p.437)

Further research is required to explore central nervous system dysfunction in relation to either HMS or DCD. However, there are known problems with HMS and DCD and ANS disorders.

Another study on HMS and DCD shows a further overlap in symptoms suffered by both conditions in relation to ANS disorders. Parents of DCD children and of typically developing children were asked questions regarding HMS, and 37 per cent of the parents of DCD children said that their children had pain plus ANS problems such as fainting, gastrointestinal symptoms and dizziness (Kirby and Davies 2007). The research needs to be repeated using a cohort of children since this study was done by parental report. Research has shown that, in children with HMS, 48 per cent of children were reported to be 'clumsy' by their parents and 36 per cent had 'poor coordination' (Adib *et al.* 2005). A further 14 per cent had a diagnosis of DCD in addition to HMS, although this study did involve children at the more severe end of the HMS spectrum; it is interesting to note the obviously related difficulties between HMS and DCD and difficulties with motor coordination. Further research is required to make connections with HMS and other learning difficulties, for example dyslexia and attention deficit disorder.

PHYSICAL EDUCATION AND SPORT

When I was cycling around France on my annual summer holiday, my attention was drawn to my knees and how they protrude 'outwards' when I am cycling, as if they are wandering off to the side instead of going forwards. Of course this movement is also initiated from my hips, but it is just an example of how my hypermobility affects me as an adult, and how this is 'normal' for me, but the way I cycle certainly looks odd and all this extra movement I have would, I reflect, have made learning to cycle more difficult for me. Indeed, it wasn't so much the oddity of the angle of my knees, but the greater challenge for me to balance and coordinate cycling which took some time to master as a child.

Upon reflection, all physical activity was difficult for me as a child, and I was an embarrassment on the sports field. I have a clear recollection of our practices for sports day in Year 2 (aged 6) where my classmates and I lined up on the sports track. I put everything into that practice race only to fall flat on my face within three metres of starting to run. This was typical. I remember the cringing embarrassment I felt on that and numerous other occasions, where my body had simply let me down because of my loose joints and poor coordination. In physical education (PE) at primary school, I could never do anything like handstands; I now understand that this would be because of my hypermobile elbows. I did not achieve my British Amateur Gymnastics Association (BAGA 4) basic level until I was 13. Most people do this much younger.

Team sports were a nightmare. Nobody wanted me in their team, a stigma which remains with me still. There is no doubt that friendships and popularity are heavily based upon one's ability in the sports field. Those who lack this ability are often shunned in other activities, because it appears they are useless. Not surprisingly, I started to skip PE by the time I was in my early teens. I would schedule my piano lessons to be during these times, if possible. Although I wasn't too bad at netball on account of my height and being a good goal shooter, I was hopeless at hockey and spent more time running (or what I do as 'running') away from the ball. I loathed athletics and was no good at swimming on account of being afraid of the water.

Although I had taken ballet classes as a young child, between the ages of 6 and 9, I recall how much longer it took me to learn to do a polka step compared to the other children, and yet I had much better facility for classical ballet than most of the children. For example, I had a good range of turnout, the aesthetics of swayback knees and a pleasing instep, despite having slightly flat feet. I gave up ballet for the first time because of a change of schooling. I left to attend a girl's school in Oxford at age 9, and started at that school in Year 5 and remained until the end of Sixth Form (Year 13). Even though I was overall very happy at this school and flourished in many ways, the stigma of my ability in sports remained a problem. I am certain it affected friendships.

LIFE AT SCHOOL

In terms of my life and performance at school, I was always a very hard worker, but whether this can be attributed to being a hypermobile, or just a personal attribute, I don't know. On reflection, I think that things such as handwriting were much harder because this returns to coordination and stamina, two things frequently lacking in hypermobile people. I still cannot do joined-up handwriting very well and now seriously fatigue when writing manually. Fortunately I can touch-type and modern technology has made an enormous difference to me. I believe that other HMS children also find typing easier than handwriting. I am not sure why I found handwriting so difficult in terms of my hypermobility because I do not have hypermobile fingers or thumbs, but then I do have very hypermobile elbows and shoulders.

LEARNING DIFFICULTIES

At school and in life in general, I have difficulties with some aspects of short-term memory retention and concentration. I have seen reference to this in other HMS literature – and there is certainly a potential link with DCD and HMS in terms of learning disorders. DCD (formerly known as dyspraxia) would be an obvious one anyway in terms of it being related to movement and coordination, something lacking in many HMS patients. Sometimes attention deficit disorder is present in adolescent HMS patients (Middleditch 2003), although research would need to be undertaken in order to prove formal learning and behavioural difficulties with HMS. As an adult I realise that my body is always distracting me which I believe still impedes my learning in classical ballet classes where I continue to struggle with long dance sequences even when I sometimes have a greater ability than others in the class. I have to concentrate more than twice as hard as the non-hypermobile person in order to organise my body, in a larger than 'normal' range of movement, especially working around pain and injuries, which are also distractions. It is all logical really – but as a child these hindrances can become stigmatic and children can be cruel to each other, and can poke fun.

Natasha, aged 11, beautifully describes her difficulties with HMS in this moving account which was conducted by interview via email. Her mother typed her responses, but no edits were made and Natasha was not led in any way. Her honesty is brutal and her responses strikingly sensitive.

Email interview with Natasha, aged 11

1. Is there anything 'good' about being hypermobile? Or for you is it all not a very good experience?

   There's absolutely nothing good about hypermobility. But I am good at doing the limbo under the tree branches I can lean further back then my friends, even more than Esme who is a dancer.

2. What are your worst symptoms or difficulties from being HMS? What helps with the symptoms/pain?

   My worse symptoms are lots of pain and getting too tired quickly. It is also affects my bladder, because I don't know when my wee comes out, so I had to wear sanitary towels all day and take medicine. I worry that other people may see I have wee'd myself. None of my friends know about the problems with my wee. My wrists are flexible and that's bad because they ache a lot which stops me being able to write or play pat-a-cake or play hit with my friends.

I learnt relaxation at Great Ormond Street [children's hospital in London] and that helps me go to sleep because I go to a happy place. My exercises are supposed to help to stop me getting pain and tired but I am not always good at remembering to do them and its boring as well. The hot wheat bags help a lot and I listen to music or watch TV to ignore the pain.

3. Is there anything that is more challenging for you at school because of being HMS?

Yes working is harder in class because I get distracted because I day dream when tired, so I get behind with my work. Answering questions is hard because they are too tricky as I am tired, and because when I am tired I can't speak clearly. Writing is hard for me because of my wrist as I get pains in my wrists. I can't keep still on the chairs because I need to move. I get tired if I have to sit on chairs for too long. Walking up the stairs can be hard because there are too many stairs. Some PE is too difficult and I feel lonely when my friends are doing PE and I can't. I get too emotional when I get bullied because I am tired and then I don't think clearly and get upset too easy. My friends sometimes leave me out, they don't do it on purpose, it's because they don't know if I am in the mood to play with them. Sometimes when I can't play there isn't anything to do, so I get bored which makes the pain worse because I can't take my mind off of it. My friends don't understand about hypermobility syndrome, I have tried explaining it and they don't listen. I get frightened of being hurt because of my EDS at school so it stops me doing things, like having fun.

Sometimes other children and teachers don't understand what I am saying so my best friend has to tell them what I have said and that is because my speech gets bad when tired. Homework can be difficult to keep on top off as I am tired after school, so I do it before lessons start in school which means I have to go to school earlier and I do homework at break time and lunch time.

4. How do the teachers help you at school?

The teachers help me with my work when I am tired. My teachers get me my splints when my wrists are aching and they get me a wheat bag to put on my back when it hurts. Sometimes they will do my writing for me. They talk to me about how I am feeling and they remind me of all the good things I can do when I am not tired. They sometimes explain to the class why I am feeling bad and they tell me to leave me alone and my friends will come and comfort me. The teachers ask me if I am hurting and check to see if I need paracetamol. When it comes to PE they talk to me and see what I can do or not. The teachers know I have a pain bag with my medicine, splints, wheat bag and Tubigrip. The teachers remind me to use my pen grips and remind not to press so hard on the paper because that makes my wrist hurt. The teachers will call mum if I am not well or really tired. The teachers in my old primary school have told the teachers at my knew school what I need to be able to go to school. Mrs Ellis helped me to be more independent at school with managing my condition. Sue [Carlyon] has helped me with my wrists by telling the other teachers I need to use a computer all the time.

5. What advice would you give to another child who had found out they had HMS?

I would tell them a different story about HMS so they wouldn't worry. I would say it will be OK, and that they aren't alone and that being with other people with HMS is a bit of fun but also a relief because they know how you feel and you don't have to explain it. I would say to them they couldn't do that much stuff like hockey and football. I would try to say positive things as well so as to not to scare them. I would tell them how much fun it is at Great Ormond Street, the rehab is fun and you get to make new friends, but it does make your body feel weird. I would tell them how to cope with the pain, going to the nurse at school, I would help them and look after them. I would tell them to ignore the pain and I would help them to ignore the pain by having some fun or go somewhere quiet so they can have a rest. I would tell someone who couldn't speak properly because of their HMS that we can stick together. If I saw that they had an accident I would lend them some spare knickers and pad. I would tell them quietly so no one else would know. I would tell the child or the teacher what was normal for us, like banging into things or having lots of bruises, I would say that they can't help it because it's our thing, its normal for us to be like that.

Natasha describes some of the other problems that might affect a child with HMS such as the weak bladder owing to tissue laxity. While I have never had to endure what Natasha has, I have always had to wake more than several times per night to use the toilet and can identify with the weak bladder. This is consistent with a study that also found 13 per cent of females and 6 per cent of males were experiencing urinary tract infections and 4 per cent of children also had urinary tract dysfunction including the urge incontinence that Natasha describes (Adib *et al.* 2005).

MANAGING MANUAL DEXTERITY – HYPERMOBILE HANDS

In terms of managing both life and school generally, Ben, aged 7, has particular difficulties with writing and managing to use cutlery owing to his severely hypermobile hands. Ben has particularly mobile fingers and thumbs, especially his index finger (see Figures 4.1, 4.2 and 4.3). This makes holding cutlery difficult, which I noticed when I watched him eating his dinner one day. Ben finds writing a challenge because of his finger hypermobility and his hand 'gets tired' when he has been writing for a while. Ben plays the violin (see Figures 4.4 and 4.5) but did not comment that he found this especially difficult, although he does not really enjoy playing the violin! Hypermobility is an advantage in instruments requiring repetitive movements, but less desirable in less frequently moved joints such as the knees and spine (Larsson *et al.* 1993).

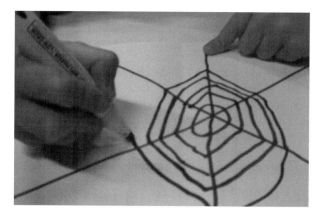

Figure 4.1: Ben, aged 7, drawing (note the finger grip on the pen)

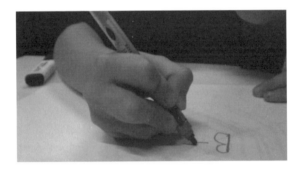

Figure 4.2: Ben, aged 7, writing (note the grip on a finer pen than in Figure 4.1)

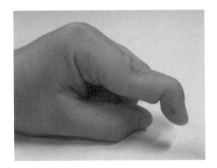

Figure 4.3: Excessive hypermobility in the index finger

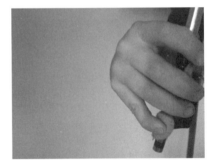

Figure 4.4: Hypermobile little finger holding a violin bow

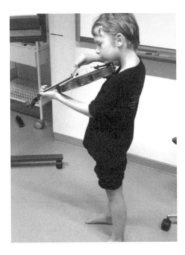

Figure 4.5: Ben, aged 7, playing his violin

Ben has particular talents in dancing and acting, which fits the general trend in those with hypermobility being drawn to the performing arts. When comparing another 7-year-old child to Ben in terms of balance, the non-hypermobile child was better, but Ben has quite hypermobile ankles and very hypermobile knees. He coped well on the flat, but not on the half-point (tip-toe) because of his hypermobility. Ben was full of a dynamic energy and was able to perform cartwheels with more elegance than his friend.

Ben did have difficulties with concentrating and is known to have dyslexia, which is not yet linked to HMS, but some of the memory and processing skills seem to have overlaps with dyspraxia or DCD. Further research is required to prove any links with dyslexia and HMS as the evidence is presently too flimsy. Ben had an assessment at school and is not thought to be DCD, but the perceived hyperactivity and poor concentration might just link in with HMS, or just that he is a lively 7-year-old boy!

Comments by Ben's mother

Ben enjoys showing people what he can do with his fingers and is happy to explain how his knees go backwards. I think I noticed Ben's hypermobile knees when he was about 4 years old and thought that he had obviously acquired his mother's hypermobility. He is starting to complain about 'aching knees' at times and is struggling to play the violin and hold his knife and fork properly. Ben was diagnosed with dyslexia last year by an educational psychologist. I was told that Ben has a poor working memory and problems with sequencing. He now attends a special school for dyslexia and dyspraxia and is working to improve his memory and organisational skills. The school's occupational therapist noticed his hypermobile fingers when he scored poorly on the fine motor and balance tasks he was asked to do. Ben is reluctant to read, write and practise his spellings. He doesn't enjoy learning the violin possibly because the lessons are heavily focused on reading musical scores. He has just been told that he will be doing football in school from next week and is absolutely dreading it. He enjoys creative play, swimming and dancing and his best thing of all is putting on shows!

MANAGING PAIN AND OTHER SYMPTOMS

Parents concerned 'parade' the children. It is quite hard to tease apart HMS until children are 12/13 years old so I usually wait to confirm diagnosis until then – unless the children have Marfan syndrome and EDS. I prefer not to label the children – some have been taken off games at school and are already ostracised. I avoid taking them off games and recommend physiotherapy unless the child is constantly fracturing or dislocating. (Professor Howard Bird, personal communication, 29 April 2010)

There is an increased risk of pain and the development of chronic pain syndromes of up to 80 per cent in children who are also hypermobile (Maillard and Payne 2010). Headaches and abdominal pains are particularly rife in HMS children: headaches often relate to muscular spasm in the neck and abdominal pain might be connected in the same way that adults' pain is – to the excessive tissue laxity of the gut. Looking at children's posture and asking how they are coping with carrying heavy bags at school are recommended. The principles of management in HMS of children are likely to be similar to adults in terms of preventing deconditioning and trying to encourage the child to continue with exercise, as long as they are strong enough to cope with the activity (Maillard and Payne 2010).

Upon serious reflection and discussion with Katherine, my physiotherapist, and with my rheumatologist, it seems possible that the prelude to my HMS becoming symptomatic was when I fractured my right leg, aged seven. We lived in a house with wooden stairs, and I was wearing socks and slipped down the last three steps with my right leg bent under me. I immediately couldn't take any weight on it. My GP didn't think I had broken it, and neither did the A&E doctors, so everyone was surprised to see a large spiral fracture of the right tibia. I was plaster-cast up to the top of my thigh for four weeks and then had a further four weeks in a knee-high plaster cast. During this time it is possible I grew a lot, and I have a recollection that my leg was set in the larger plaster cast in my maximal hyper-extension. As a result, the right leg has remained not only shorter than the left, but there is considerable more hypermobility in the right knee and hip compared to the left leg (see Figure 4.6). My right foot also ended up being one size different to the left, until adulthood. I was not given physiotherapy following this injury and did not walk properly for over a year. I don't think that the right leg has ever functioned properly again since this time, which has had a significant impact on my symptoms and has contributed to a mild scoliosis and ultimately to back pain, which began when I was 17.

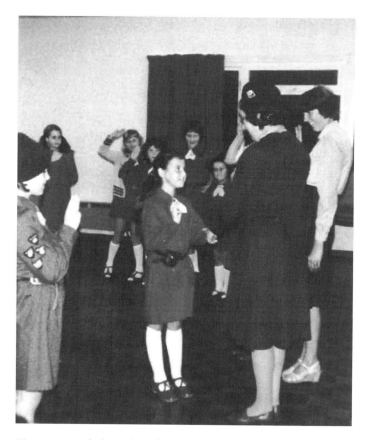

Figure 4.6: Isobel, aged 8. If this photograph had been taken from the side, hypermobility of the knees would be extremely obvious. Even here the muscle bulk is different in the right and left calves

Since I had all the hallmarks of HMS prior to this event – including the delayed walking, poor motor control and coordination and was always labelled as an 'awkward child' in a movement capacity – it is unfortunate that I was not further investigated because observation of my standing and movement would have highlighted that there were problems. I do recall my leg hurting, but I was generally very stoical and I suspect that I didn't complain as much as I could have done. It was accepted the leg would continue to be painful for a while following removal of the plaster cast and I suspect I just got used to it and worked around it. My message would therefore be that if you have a child who has some of the hallmarks discussed in this chapter, including pain, not to accept this as a normal state of affairs and to seek medical intervention. I believe that if I had been properly rehabilitated following my leg fracture, I might not have gone on to develop quite so many other symptoms, pain and difficulty later on in life. Early intervention in this medical condition is highly advantageous in making it a much more manageable condition (Knight and Bird 2010).

CONCLUSION

This chapter discussed the following points:

- Bottom shuffling and delayed walking might be indicative suggestions of joint hypermobility.

- Clumsiness and lack of muscular control and poor coordination might indicate hypermobility.

- There are links with HMS and DCD.

- Children might find handwriting and fine motor coordination more difficult.

- Children's pain management should be addressed early and exercise programmes carefully paced.

- Early intervention and medical management is likely to have a much more desirable effect and improved outcome.

CHAPTER 5

Adolescents and HMS

A Smile to Hide the Pain

I put on a smile to hide my own pain,
But sometimes the tears fall like heavy rain,
I tell the doctors how I feel,
But I don't think they know it's real.
I want to run and have some fun,
Just to enjoy the midday sun,
I know that people think it's all in your head,
But when I do too much I spend a week in bed,
I would love to go back to school,
To play around and be the fool,
I wish one day it would all go away,
So I could start again and go out to play,
I remember things before my pain,
Now a distant memory and all in vain.

(© Kate, aged 16, in Newson 2010)

Kate's powerful poem clearly illustrates what it means to be adolescent and have HMS, and how it robs people of fun and an enjoyable quality of life. At a lecture given at the University of Hertfordshire on 1 July 2010, Professor Rodney Grahame, a leading expert in HMS, talked about how patients with HMS were often high achievers and highly motivated, cut down in their prime. I was particularly struck by that comment, because it is so true. Already by adolescence I was experiencing problems which are now clearly linked to HMS, and by early adulthood my life was becoming significantly affected by my HMS symptoms. I also particularly liked the possibility of being a high achiever – perhaps I can aspire to that, while being highly motivated I can certainly recognise.

Preliminary research looking at an adolescent dance population and differences between HMS dancers and non-HMS dancers in terms of perfectionism scores showed that HMS dancers scored significantly higher (Knight 2009a), so perhaps this tallies with Professor Grahame's observations. One explanation for the high perfectionism scores might link in to over-compensations to control a large range of movement in an 'out of control' body, but this is speculative. It might simply be that these dancers are more ambitious!

> It's not fair that I can't be normal like my mates. It's your fault for giving me HMS and my life is crap! (Adolescent boy displaying anger at his mother)

Most teenagers go through a time whereby their limbs and their bodies in general seem 'out of control' during the turbulence of puberty. It is a universally difficult time when attitudes change, independence is sought and rebellion is in the air. I became more aware of my hypermobility in my teenage years and had terrible growing pains, particularly in my knees. HMS teenagers are more likely to experience growing pains but these and muscle spasms may also relate to unaccustomed exercise and overuse of weakened muscles (Maillard and Murray 2003; Maillard and Payne 2010).

In my teenage years my ballet teacher told me that I had swayback knees. I understood that there was a problem with my knees because first position of the feet was hard to achieve as it is difficult to enable the heels to touch. There are different schools of thought as to whether teachers should allow for the gap or close the gap. Personally, I think that leaving a small heel gap is preferable just so that the dancer might attempt to engage their adductor muscles, which are frequently weak in hypermobile dancers. I remember finding *ronds de jambe* (see Chapter 10) very difficult because the feet have to pass through first position of the feet. It is hard for hypermobile people to not go to the end of their range and soften limbs into what for other people would be a normal neutral line.

Outside of the ballet studio, all my other HMS 'symptoms' started to flare up in my teenage years. I had asthma and hay fever – I wouldn't have classed myself as seriously asthmatic, but I did need an inhaler infrequently, in the summer, or if I had a cold. I would have intermittent episodes of constipation and/or diarrhoea, which are IBS related, and would need regular visits to the bathroom during the night. Gynaecologically I experienced severe menstrual pain almost from first menarche. There were years of hot water bottles, needing to go to sick bay at school and strong, but ineffective, painkillers. In my late teenage years I went on the contraceptive pill, but now I know that this would have aggravated joint pain. Lower back pain started weeks before my eighteenth birthday and has remained an almost permanent fixture. There was regular soft-tissue trauma – most frequently minor tears to my calf muscles on an almost weekly basis – mainly because my calves were overworking at the expense of other inefficient muscular groups. I started to experience fatigue: I remember often feeling wiped out, but seldom refreshed, from sleep, even if I did sleep well, which was rarely the case. At least I was lucky not to dislocate any joints!

> The evolution of the symptom complex associated with JHS untreated can be seen as a slowly developing crescendo of painful short-lived soft tissue traumatic incidents, occurring sequentially and building up momentum of severity, frequency and duration over time. Slow and often incomplete healing of individual lesions results in a blurring of their margins, so that pain transforms from discontinuous to continuous, from recurrent acute to sub-acute and ultimately, to chronic. (Grahame 2010, p.29)

Two factors that reinforce this are a lack of effective medication and an avoidance of movement as it becomes increasingly painful (Grahame 2010). Although I was not avoiding movement as such by adolescence because I danced, I avoided sport, but this was mainly because I wasn't good at it. In Chapter 6, I clearly explain how I did deteriorate owing to eventual movement 'kinesiophobia', phobia of movement when I eventually stopped all forms of exercise, including ballet.

Physicians advocate the importance of continued exercise, sport and movement in HMS patients of all ages, and it is essential to reach the adolescent population before they totally stop exercise and completely decondition: 'hypermobile adolescents must be encouraged to take regular exercise or play sport. The benefits of physical activity include improving cardiovascular fitness, improvements in muscle strength and control, coordination and a feeling of wellbeing' (Middleditch 2010, p.174). The important thing is for adolescents to find something they enjoy doing because they are much more likely to keep playing the sport or attend classes. There might be some issues over playing very high contact sports such as rugby for the most severely hypermobile. In the performing arts, hypermobility can be desirable and many dancers, gymnasts, acrobats and musicians are drawn to their art based upon their effortless range of movement (McCormack *et al.* 2004). Dancers are discussed in greater detail in Chapter 10.

Some HMS adolescents, however, will be more severely affected than others. Alex tells her story.

Because of my family history I kind of knew I had it so didn't go to the doctors for stuff and only got diagnosed when I was 15 (I'm 16 now), and I thought things were normal that weren't like dislocations. I started sixth form but stopped going in December last year because I couldn't cope with getting ready to go to school every day or all the walking around, sitting in lessons, writing, etc., and because I was always so achy and tired I found it really hard to concentrate and didn't complete any of my class or homework for the whole 4 months, which was really upsetting because I wanted to do well, so I thought the best thing to do was to take at least the rest of the year out to try and get things under control so I could seriously look at going back into education. I am so much happier for being out of school and am making good progress with my physio now and everybody says it was a good decision, even my doctors!

I struggle with washing a lot because I have to do that every day but I saw an occupational therapist which made things easier because I have a seat in my shower now. I have a lot of trouble with balance and proprioception. I'm not great at walking but I don't have to do any a lot at the moment, and I have really rubbish stamina. To help with things I take anti-inflammatory for tendonitis and pain, acid blockers for reflux, and very low dose of anti-depressants for chronic pain and to encourage me to sleep better which helps a little bit with fatigue.

The best things for me have been physio which I have done over about 5 years and pacing. The most difficult thing for me is not doing loads of stuff when I feel better than normal. I also plan everything I am going to do for the next two weeks and sometimes further so I can make sure I don't overdo things but also that I am doing enough. I spread things I need to do out that are difficult, for example I don't eat my lunch all at once because otherwise my jaws really hurt. I also make sure I have plenty of time to do things so when I get tired I can take things slowly and don't have to rush. I am very reliant on my mum and sister though. (Alex, aged 16)

MANAGEMENT STRATEGIES

Fatigue is experienced by most HMS patients and there is more about this in Chapters 2 and 7. Alex's story is an extreme account of how HMS can seriously affect quality of life and how navigating school was a great challenge for her. Adolescents need support with pacing their day and might need help in carrying heavy school bags, which might aggravate dislocations, or subluxations, not to mention increasing fatigue. A good backpack is one way to support students and avoid undue stress on upper limbs. Correcting sitting postures and arranging support for students can help them to manage prolonged sitting. The use of pens with 'thick grip' and adaptable keyboards are other strategies that adolescents can use to support them at school (see Middleditch 2003).

Adolescents from the HMSA Forum have the following things to say:

I found out I had HMS about two months ago. My knees started to give way when I ran and hurt a lot. My mum took me to the doctors and they said I had damaged cartilages and that it would go away, that was about 9 months ago and they have started to get worse. But now I know that it was because of my HMS. Now I cannot do any gym at school and I have a lift key as I can no longer use the stairs. It's hard having HMS as a kid because while all your friends are out running about and having a laugh you can't as it's too sore. Also kids automatically assume that if their knees are a bit sore they have HMS which can be a nuisance. And some teachers treat you as though you are disabled and can't walk.

For many years I have had health problems, feeling weak and my muscles ached most of the time. I did have a lot of energy and even went to dancing classes. I loved going out for bike rides and going to the shops with my mum and dad. All that stopped three years ago when the weakness worsened and the pain in my legs became unbearable. Painkillers did not work and I had to go to bed and rest. The only thing that helped was when my mum applied 'Deep Heat' to my legs. My mum and dad saw many doctors over these three years, none of whom gave any answers. Some suggested that we were making it up. In May 1999 mum asked for a second opinion away from our area and we were sent to Manchester Children's Hospital. We saw two doctors who diagnosed that I had hypermobility syndrome. At last I knew that someone believed me.

In June 1999, I was lucky to be seen by Professor Grahame who was in Glasgow for a conference. Also there was Dr Ferrell of Glasgow Royal. They were both nice to me and my mum which made a change. I am now getting physiotherapy to help me, but as I am in my first year at High School, it is quite hard. I still do not have any energy and even going to the shops is difficult and leaves me feeling tired. Some days I can feel quite ill. I just want to be like my friends doing everyday things. I worry at times about what kind of job I will do when I leave school as I know there are many jobs I could not manage.

Hopefully with the physiotherapy I will gain some strength but I do find the exercises hard to do every day on top of homework. Sometimes I get a bit down.

Hi I am 15 years old and I have had HMS for about 5 years. It all started with a pain in my left knee and I had surgery and physiotherapy but nothing changed and from then on it has progressed and most of my body is hypermobile and most of my joints easily dislocate. This year I started my GCSE's and took PE because I was part of the school Hockey, rounder and tennis teams and I really enjoyed sport but my HMS has got so bad I have been forced to give it all up and I am now spending most of my time on crutches. I was gutted! And unfortunately I have got to wait for my bones to stop growing before I have corrective operations. Although HMS has totally changed my life I have always had loads of support from my family, friends and especially my boyfriend. And the HMSA website has helped me loads and now I know I am not alone and lots of people know what I am going through. Thank you!

I am 13 I have been diagnosed with HMS for about 4 months now I started having pains in my lower back then about a month or so it spread all over my body I even started pains in my head! I can't even count how many times my mum took me to the GP and them saying it will go in a week! But it didn't. My mum started taking me to hospital about 2 times a week and begging them to tell us what was wrong with me. But no answers. My whole family and all the doctors I have seen have thought I was making it all up to avoid school and that made me so upset then after about a year I was referred to Great Ormond Street hospital and they diagnosed me with benign joint hypermobility and now I'm doing physio. I'm relieved I know what is wrong with me because I have missed months of school and really want to go back full time but I know I won't manage it all. I really want to promote awareness of this because I don't want people to go through what I have gone through with people thinking you have made it all up.

A mother of two children with HMS makes the following comments to conclude this chapter.

As a mum of two children with HMS/EDS, I find I act as a coach, counsellor and problem solver. With the right help children with HMS/EDS do not need to be disadvantaged in any aspect of normal life.

Teaching your child about exercising and remaining strong can be a battle, particularly towards the end of term when all children are becoming 'tired', but our children in particular become 'fatigued'. I sometimes wonder if I am being too harsh with regards to exercising, attendance at school and encouragement to use pain management and pacing strategies but then I look at myself and see the damage that 'non-management' of HMS/EDS can cause: a shortened career, becoming dependent on partners or children, reduced family income, increase in mental health problems and social isolation. When I look at these factors I know that being proactive is the right thing to do.

This doesn't mean I won't validate their feelings, frustrations and experiences of living with a long term condition such as HMS/EDS. I do! My own experiences of being made to feel I was neurotic will never allow me to dismiss the effects of HMS/EDS. I make sure that I listen to how they feel and then take the time to explain that they need to overcome the pain and fatigue and why.

As our children spend the majority of their time at school I strongly believe that parents and teachers need to work together to ensure that children with HMS/EDS are given access to all spectrums of the school curriculum. This may mean having a meeting prior to starting school and 'teaching the teachers' about the HMS and the need to allow the child to function within the school. Just allowing teachers to understand that there is a need for children to be able to fidget, access toilets or First Aid when needed, recognising that a child appearing to not being paying attention may be fatigued or in pain can all help to enhance the child's experiences at school. In fact school can be an effective pain management tool, as it offers many distractions!

Schools may need to bring in an OT to ensure that children who are struggling with writing due to pain in their fingers and wrists are assessed and advised of solutions to reduce the pain. This could mean simple solutions such as different pen grips, correction of how a child holds a pen or as in other cases such as my daughter's needing to move onto working with the aid of IT equipment. The need to problem solve shouldn't be ignored for any given difficulty that the child faces. The provision of a locker at school and a spare set of text books at home lessens the need for our children to carry heavy bags, especially on PE days.

I do believe that PE is essential to a HMS/EDS child. While not all children can cope with contact sports, PE teachers can and should offer a modified PE programme. This could involve improving core strength or proprioception. The need for a physio to come into school to assess a child may need to be considered especially if the child is really struggling in PE lessons, which really would highlight a need for some form of intervention. Discussing pain management strategies with teachers, nurses, SENCOs and having a written pain management plan for all to refer to is extremely helpful. Most schools will allow ice packs, wheat bags, splints and pain medication to be held with the school nurse. Teaching children to be able to manage their injuries themselves will give them a sense of confidence and increase their chance of staying within the school environment instead of being sent home or to A&E. (Donna Wicks, HMSA Medical Liaison Officer and mother of two)

CHAPTER 6

Pain Management and Adults and HMS

The Noise!

The noise. The noise!
Imagine the neighbourhood dog never shuts-up,
The perpetual cry of a hungry baby.
Continuous road-digging or a wailing car alarm.
This is the terrible sound of chronic pain.
It is often so loud that I can hardly hear a normal human conversation.

To match the pain that I am experiencing I might down six vodka and
  tonics,
Burn myself with an iron, rip my skin, down some morphine, or
  destroy a room.
There is a roaring fire inside me that wants me to grind the hot coals
  of pain to powder.
If I could scream loud enough, the road outside would rip apart.
The guts of the earth would embowel and be strewn over the street.

A drill bores into my lower back.
The pain here is so intensely focussed I could nail it.
The pain in my pelvis is blunt. Broad. Flat. Dull. Laboured. Heavy.
  Grey.
Two areas each the size of stones feel sore and tender. They
  resonate.
The pain in my middle pulls me down like the weight of a rock.
Like an injured animal I crawl, dragging this all with me everywhere
  I go.

(© *Isobel Knight 2009b*)

Chapter 3 explored the diagnosis of HMS. Given the complexity of diagnosis and the possibility of delayed and/or misdiagnosis of HMS, there may be many people who have endured years of pain without fully understanding why this might be. The overriding complaint in connection with HMS is usually pain, yet one of the hardest things to explain is that the pain might have started without any particular incident, injury or trauma, but once it is there it rarely goes away (Grahame 2003, 2009a, 2009b; Keer 2003).

In my own case I recall the beginning of chronic lower back pain two weeks before my eighteenth birthday. I had just done a ballet exam and wondered whether I had pushed myself too hard. I remembered returning home from class with a blunt but localised pain in my lower back. Initially I tried resting, mild painkillers and exercise modification under the guidance of my ballet teacher. After two weeks with no major improvements I saw my GP, who referred me for my first sessions of physiotherapy. The physiotherapist I saw was not familiar with dance-related injuries, let alone widespread hypermobility (I suspect), and suggested that my pain was resulting from sacroiliac strain. I was treated accordingly with ultrasound and gentle hands-on manipulation. I had six sessions of physiotherapy and for a period of about four years my pain remained intermittent, worse during menstruation (Bird 2004, 2007b). Other factors such as growing pains, regular night cramps, very frequent soft-tissue trauma and a history of fractures would have suggested that I had HMS. I now suspect that the pain began because of overuse, a common phenomenon in HMS, and hinging at that level of my spine. What I urgently needed all along (since adolescence, if not before), and did not adequately receive until two years ago, was remedial physiotherapy and Pilates to address my lack of core stability. My story in terms of my pain starting without major incident is far from uncommon within the HMS community.

ACUTE PAIN

Acute pain is caused by an obvious trauma, accident or incident. Examples include burning oneself on an iron, spraining an ankle and falling down and dislocating a joint (something that can happen regularly to HMS patients). The pain may be severe and sudden, and may heal and go away over a period of time, but the pain is a warning signal that there is a problem and that you need to take action. However, there is an end to acute pain and it does respond to analgesia, rest, ice/heat, manipulation/ massage, as required (Nicholas *et al.* 2005).

CHRONIC PAIN

Compared to its acute counterpart, chronic pain does not go away and might remain indefinitely. 'Chronic pain is usually insidious, superimposing itself on the pattern of often widespread musculoskeletal pain that went before' (Grahame 2009b, p.430). Chronic pain may be defined as pain that has lasted persistently for more than three months' duration, and often much longer than that. The pain might start without a very obvious incident or resultant trauma; however, *nociceptive pain* is pain whereby tissue damage persists and leads to pain. Examples of this might include cancer, post-operative pain and arthritis. *Neuropathic pain* may be described as shooting pain, or hot pain, due to damage or injury to the nerves. Shingles is a good example of neuropathic pain. Neuropathic pain results in changes to the central nervous system where the memory of the pain remains, and the body continues to respond to pain signals that no longer usefully alert the body to pain. This is how pain becomes chronic, and it can remain unrelenting, often unresponsive to analgesia (Grahame 2009b; Nicholas *et al.* 2005).

Chronic pain can share elements of both nociceptive and neuropathic pain and that there might be an unclear distinction between both types of pain. Chronic pain is the result of the body continuing to experience and perceive pain long after an event and the pain signals remain active. In the long term this results in changes to the central nervous system. Unfortunately the reasons for the resultant change in pain response are not fully understood, but ultimately the patient has to cope with and manage them. This is where good pain management is vital (Nicholas *et al.* 2005).

In HMS, chronic pain is often made worse by any kind of movement and so patients increasingly start to avoid movement as a management strategy. This is 'kinesiophobia' or movement phobia. Avoiding movement leads to muscle deconditioning, which is detrimental to patients whose joints are already unstable. It is no surprise that the less an HMS patient moves and the more they decline to function, the worse their pain becomes, and this in turn leads to a loss of independence

(Grahame 2009b). By the time I was sent to a pain management clinic, I had long since given up dancing and any other form of exercise. I had gained a large amount of weight, was in more pain than before and was barely working. Like many other HMS patients, my symptoms had often been missed and dismissed, I had not always received adequate support from the medical profession and I experienced feelings of anger and resentment (Grahame 2009a; Harding 2003; Simmonds 2003).

SENSITISED SENSATION AND PAIN AMPLIFICATION

Patients with chronic pain often develop increased sensation and amplification in their greatest areas of pain. This is caused by changes to the nociceptive neurons, which are the neurons found in skin, joint, muscle, fascia and tendon tissues. Eventually the nociceptive neurons change in response to trauma or further inflammation and gradually their sensitivity to pain increases over time. This can be difficult to cope with because the increased pain makes sufferers want to do less in order to protect the area, or they become more anxious that they have reinjured the area or made it worse. I sometimes find it hard to distinguish between pain that is alerting me to a new problem and pain that is there routinely. This is particularly difficult with pelvic pain, but when I have ended up in A&E in acute pain, my instinct has been right and there has been something different causing my pain to rocket. I am thinking of endometriosis in this instance. At other times, my lower back can 'hurt like hell' for no particular reason, but I know that there is nothing sinister going on and that gentle movement, painkillers where necessary and Bowen or exercise will help to relieve it, even if this takes several days. In chronic pain terms, this might be called a flare up. It is still a problem to cope with, and sometimes when my pain is amplified in this way, it is like being shouted at loudly. This makes it difficult to concentrate and manage other people or stressful and challenging situations. Although I am usually a calm and smiley person, there are times when I want to yell and shout at other people because the pain is drowning me out. Even when someone is experiencing amplified chronic pain flare ups, it is still invisible to other people, and perhaps only a shortened temper would indicate what the sufferer is experiencing.

HOW CAN YOU MANAGE THIS?

The rest of this chapter explores pain management, and also looks at aspects such as goal-setting, relaxation and types of medication and dealing with pain in a psychological capacity. I think that you have to be strong about communicating your needs, and Chapter 9 will go into this in more detail.

Chronic pain will improve if it is managed effectively. I have learned over time what helps me when my lower back flares up and the pain becomes more amplified. My family usually know if I am not too good just by looking at my face and are supportive by doing things like making me hot water bottles as I find heat helps. They speak more quietly to me and understand if I am not very chatty and need more rest and quiet time.

At work I usually try to do more mundane tasks or tasks that I normally enjoy because it makes me feel psychologically better if I have achieved something. Having understanding colleagues and a sympathetic and supportive line manager also help. If in the middle of a flare up, I wouldn't actively choose to do something very difficult or a high cerebral task because I am less likely to succeed, then feel depressed and stressed, all of which are likely to increase the pain. Moving about more at work helps me and I am more restless when I am in a great deal of pain. I also appreciate being left alone or to work in peace and quiet when in more pain. Other strategies that can help are having a brief rest at lunch time or taking a taxi home because public transport is just one bridge too far for me. Lovely people giving me lifts home is also appreciated. All the little things and general acts of kindness make so much difference. Someone making you a cup of tea, listening to you and then making you laugh makes pain management possible. I find having a cat very therapeutic and, although I cannot take him to work, he appears to be very sensitive to me when I am in more pain – perhaps animal intuition, and for that I am very grateful.

PAIN MANAGEMENT – ANALGESIA

When I finally attended a four-week residential pain management course at a central London hospital, my back pain had become less dehabilitating than it had been (see p.96). By this point I had been in pain for ten years. I had seen numerous experts including osteopaths, orthopaedic surgeons and neurosurgeons. An MRI scan had revealed a minor disc prolapse and disc degeneration, which is hastened in HMS patients. I also had severe pelvic pain, which was diagnosed as endometriosis (see Chapter 8), which caused my back pain to amplify significantly because of further irritation caused by the same nerve endings in the lumbar and pelvic region.

In the end I was sent to see pain management consultants because mainline analgesia or pain relief had largely been unsuccessful. This is often the case in terms of chronic pain, but it is important to mention the types of medications available, and that there are several strands or branches of drugs that do different things (see Table 6.1).

Table 6.1: Drug group examples

Opiates	NSAIDS	Tricyclics	SSRIs	Anti-convulsants	Tran-quillisers	Miscel-laneous
Morphine	Ibuprofen	Amitriptyline	Fluoxetine	Gabapentin	Diazepam	Alternative
Sevredol	Diclofenac	Dosulepin	(Prozac)		(Valium)	medicine
Dihydrocodeine	Mefenamic		Sertraline			Cannabis
(DF-118)	acid (Ponstan)		Duloxetine			
Co-proxamol	Aspirin					
Co-codamol	Paracetamol					

The theory is that one drug from each group is probably the most effective in the case of acute injury or post-operative pain, but in terms of chronic pain management it is important to weigh up benefits against side effects. There are only a certain amount of receptors (which absorb the medication) in each of us; some drugs are long-acting and some are short-acting.

Each drug group carries different side effects. For example, some side effects of opiates are constipation, delusions, sickness and drowsiness. Some side effects of non-steroidal anti-inflammatory drugs (NSAIDs) are stomach problems as they can cause stomach ulcers and heart disease: some NSAIDs (such as COX-2 inhibitors) now damage some of the body's enzymes that protect the heart. NSAIDs only work most effectively for acute pain, or straight after an injury, so are more unhelpful for chronic pain. Side effects of tricyclics can be palpitations, dry mouth, drowsiness and weight gain, and take two weeks to work, so you get maximum side effects if you stop them too quickly. Side effects of selective serotonin reuptake inhibitors (SSRIs) might inhibit the analgesic effect of Tramadol and Codeine (Martin-Santos, Bulbena and Crippa 2010, p.58). Side effects of Gabapentin can be excessive sleepiness. Side effects of tranquillisers can be addiction – they are more addictive than cocaine!

Alternative medicine is not formally tested (as yet) or evidence-based medicine. Nicotine is known to be counterproductive in patients with chronic pain and can work against the body in any good you might be trying to do, for example more exercise.

While analgesia is certainly beneficial in acute pain and perhaps for flare ups with chronic pain, its efficacy is less assured overall for chronic pain, and the management of chronic pain becomes different.

Complementary and alternative medicine

Many patients in pain will have tried not only a conventional and orthodox western medicine, but also complementary and alternative medicines with varying degrees of success. Further information about complementary medicine is in Chapter 11.

MANAGEMENT OF CHRONIC PAIN

For my own condition, a number of approaches had already been attempted by another hospital pain team. I was initially given a course of acupuncture which unfortunately did not help me, but I know of other patients who have benefited from this. I was also given use of a TENS machine. The Transcutaneous Electrical Nerve Stimulator (TENS) involves the location of four sticky pads applied around the site of the pain which deliver electronic signals in pulses and various different strengths of signals. The theory behind the TENS is that it is meant to scramble the pain messages sent by one's own nervous system. Although the TENS did not actually work for me, it did at least distract the unrelenting pain signals for a while.

I had already by this point exhausted many of the mainstream medications including opioids. Following the TENS, I was put on two different types of drugs. The first drug was Gabapentin, which is aimed at neuropathic pain, and the second drug was Dosulepin, an antidepressant, but prescribed more to aid sleep rather than because I was especially depressive (at this time). Unfortunately I did not tolerate Dosulepin and suffered from tachycardia (fast heart rate) so I stopped this drug. In the end, Gabapentin also did nothing for my neuropathic pain despite being on 3000mg per day.

At the start of this new drug regime, I was asked to restart exercise, but given very little guidance about how to do this. I believe that this is a common problem for HMS and other people experiencing chronic pain. I was told I had to do the exercise as part of the treatment. I didn't swim at this time, but could swim with floats, and my local swimming pool had a hydrotherapy pool which was much warmer than a normal pool and had adjustable depth and bubbles. At the age of 25, I attended their sessions for 'disabled/elderly/injured' patients. I remember that my 'best friend' at hydrotherapy was a man called Bill, who was 78. Sometimes I enjoyed being in this great big bath of a swimming pool, but otherwise I felt very angry about the pain I was in and I sometimes smashed my back against the wall of the pool because I just wanted it all to go away.

At the same time I started to do Pilates, which I hoped would give me the abdominal muscles I had always dreamed of and, more technically, improve my core stability so that my painful back might have more muscular support. Joseph Pilates created this method based on allowing people to optimise their health and physical wellbeing and correcting imbalances and weaknesses (Friedman and Eisen 1980). I attended often 'large' classes and, despite telling the teacher about my back pain, it was probably impossible for her to seriously address my problems at a more individual level. As a result my pain was regularly worse and I often experienced systemic musculoskeletal pain which I now know is linked in with HMS and the fact that my body was so deconditioned that I need to recruit much larger groups of muscles in order to stabilise one small area (Grahame 2009b; Keer 2003).

The resultant fatigue that is sometimes overlooked in patients with HMS and chronic pain can be incredibly debilitating. Partly, perhaps, because of their continued experience of extra movement and regularly being in pain, people with HMS are more likely to experience fatigue and flu-like symptoms.

After terminating Gabapentin, my next option included trying lumbar epidural injections for the pain. Having an epidural is a surgical procedure which requires fasting. A canula is inserted in the back of the hand in case extra fluids are required during the procedure. The injection is administered in an operating theatre, and you are fully conscious. I felt quite nervous sitting under the bright theatre light and seeing the heart rate monitor, oxygen bottles and other surgical implements at hand in case things went wrong. The first thing that happened was that my back was painted with a yellow antiseptic fluid called Betadine. When having an epidural the area is sterilised to minimise infection. I was asked to curl up in a ball so that my spine was at optimal flexion and so that the consultant anaesthetist could locate the site of pain. The local anaesthetic was actually more painful than the epidural, and I remember it stinging as it went in. After that the epidural was prepared while the local anaesthetic took effect. What I remember most is feeling a lot of pressure as they inserted quite a long needle into my spine, though I never looked. Once it was all over I was wheeled to recovery.

Initially it felt like I had been kicked in the back, but after a while I did notice a brief improvement. Despite having a few of these injections, the pain returned, or would still flare up at times. Patients with HMS do not respond very well to local anaesthesia including epidural injections, and dental anaesthesia is not always effective in providing adequate pain relief: the effect of the anaesthetic remains much shorter in patients with HMS (Hakim *et al.* 2005). Quite why this is the case remains unsolved; however, if you are diagnosed with HMS, you should tell your dentist and hospital consultants in case you need local anaesthesia so that they can arrange a more continuous supply (for example, of Lidocaine).

We know that people with EDS hypermobility don't get the full local anaesthetic effect. We know that it is not a complete lack of effect, partial lack of effect, reduced effect and that duration of effect is also reduced, and we know that, of patients with the syndrome who were asked if they could remember incidents where local anaesthetic was not effective, 2/3 (of 200 patients surveyed) said yes. The only theory as to why was put forward by the group who first reported this and they thought it was due to the presence of lax and stretchy tissue that the anaesthetic escaped more quickly. Most dentists will give more anaesthesia when you inform them you have HMS. (Professor Rodney Grahame, personal communication, 20 October 2010)

ATTENDING A RESIDENTIAL PAIN MANAGEMENT COURSE

I attended a residential pain management course following the largely unsuccessful epidural injections. The course took place at a central London hospital over a four-week period. There were eight of us in the group, and over eighty years of pain between us, with many of us experiencing pain for over ten years. One critical statement in one of our first lectures from a consultant anaesthetist was that 'pain does not equal damage'. It was because of that profound statement that I restarted classical ballet classes following a nine-year gap.

Even though my pain was somewhat improved by this time, largely due to having Bowen therapy, there were many benefits to attending the course, the first being a return to exercise. I clearly remember some of the other group members finding the physical aspect of the course a great challenge, but because I was one of the youngest and thus less deconditioned, I coped well with the exercise regime. The psychological and emotional impact was much tougher for me than I had bargained for (see p.104).

EXERCISE – STRETCHING

As already mentioned, hypermobile people decondition and lose muscle tone quickly and often stop exercising because of injury or resultant pain. They often display considerable joint instability, reduced muscle strength and endurance, poor proprioception and vulnerability to injury (Simmonds 2003, p.111). People with HMS do not tolerate overuse or repetition well, partly as a result of a lack of muscular endurance, which can lead to further injury. Hypermobile people might be less able to tolerate repetition because the muscles are working harder to control an extra range of movement, which might explain why their muscles fatigue sooner than in non-hypermobiles, and they feel tired (Keer *et al.* 2003; McCormack *et al.* 2004; Roussel *et al.* 2009; Ruemper 2008).

Potential theories to explain patients' behaviour mentions that their poor muscle tone makes it difficult for them to sustain postures (Keer *et al.* 2003). In particular, patients with HMS seem to exhibit poor muscular endurance, which might explain their inability to sustain positions, hence the 'fidgeting' (Middleditch 2003; Simmonds 2003). Nevertheless it is crucial that HMS patients develop muscular endurance to provide support to their lax joints and to improve posture and therefore reduce injury.

A physiotherapist describes the patients she sees at the INPUT Pain Management Centre as having a quality of 'grace and drape', which she also observes in the family of the hypermobile patients, which would certainly relate to HMS being a genetic condition (Harding 2003; Raff and Byers 1996; Simpson 2006). The physiotherapist describes how the HMS patients behave in stretch class: 'most patients look rather unhappy with the stretches; however, those with joint hypermobility seem to love it and are practically purring afterwards!' (Harding 2003, p.155). The relief that HMS patients gain from stretching might be linked to relief of feelings of muscle stiffness which is related to the condition and stretching might relieve growing pains in adolescents (Keer 2003; Middleditch 2003). However, it might be that people with HMS enjoy stretch class, simply because they are good at it.

Apart from the academic reasons, I enjoyed stretch because I was good at stretching. There is a relief, a bit like scratching an itch, to be gained from stretch, and I think that is what physiotherapists mean about relief from muscle stiffness, plus it seems to help with muscle fatigue. I still enjoy collapsing into a big forward flexion stretch after working my upper back and shoulders in Pilates, much to the instructors' annoyance!

Some medical professionals think that hypermobile people do not need to stretch, but there is a difference in the hypermobile person going to the extreme end of range in their loosest joints, to stretching areas where they have less flexibility. Most hypermobile areas have some quite stiff segments, for example in the spine, to compensate for the hypermobile areas. This is structurally necessary in order to protect the hypermobile areas. It is the less flexible areas that really would benefit from stretching, whereas someone who already has very flexible hips or hamstrings would not need to increase flexibility where they already have plenty of movement. It is all common sense really and a stretch programme is usually created by an expert, such as a physiotherapist. The programme I followed incorporated stretches all over the body including the hands and feet, but nothing should cause pain to the extent one needs to hold one's breath or screw up the face. For further advice about treatments and physiotherapy, see Chapter 11.

EXERCISE – CIRCUITS

The second exercise aspect at the pain management course I attended involved what was known as 'circuits'. In the absence of a structured gym, circuits was an adapted set of exercises that could be done anywhere, including your own home. Exercises were designed to incorporate all aspects of physical exercise including a cardiovascular element (Simmonds 2010). The following exercises are examples and are not recommended as a self-exercise programme. Do not try them out; instead seek advice from your own GP, physiotherapist or gym instructor.

Circuits involved (some examples):

- running on the spot

- going on an exercise bike

- running up and down stairs

- push ups

- arm circles

- tummy lifts

- leg lifts

- stand ups (from a chair).

I found circuits to be much harder than stretch, because my cardiovascular fitness is quite poor and because running and any element of speed require coordination and muscular endurance, and I am not very good at it! I am sure there are other readers nodding their heads at this point. I think that perhaps hypermobility, speed and agility do not go very well together, but that is a personal opinion.

For many of us on the pain management course, the experience of both exercise and chronic pain had not been a good one. We could identify with starting ambitious gym programmes that failed after about day three because the radical increase in exercise caused our pain to flare up massively and our deconditioned bodies were not ready for the intensity of a gym programme. Even walking has huge implications for the hypermobile person. The physiotherapist who started working me in 2008 made the following observations about hypermobile people walking: 'It is incredible watching people with HMS walk. Their movement patterns are not efficient. They loll around and hang into the hips, swaying side to side and are not moving "over" the hips' (Katherine Watkins, personal communication, 22 April 2010). Given the complexities of walking, it is perhaps easy to see where anything requiring more speed is likely to cause even greater chaos and an increased pain in bodies where there is a huge ROM, a lack of muscular endurance and possible deconditioning, hence HMS patients' poor experiences of gyms.

The circuit exercises in the pain management course were intended as a way back into exercise, rather than a means to an end. Table 6.2 shows what I managed to achieve during the four weeks I was in attendance. It has to be acknowledged that my fitness was better than some people's on the course, but nevertheless progress was evident. Remember also that I wanted to go back to classical ballet classes as my 'return to exercise' (Knight 2010a).

Table 6.2: Isobel Knight's pre- and post-course readings

	Pre-course	Last day
Date	29 August 2006	21 September 2006
5 minute walk (metres)	441	479
1 minute of stand ups	23	35
1 minute of stairs	118	136

Other pain management courses will have their own variations of exercises. Chapters 10 and 11 address ways in which you can begin exercise. Remember to get consent from your own GP or medical expert before you begin any exercise programmes. Despite the types of things that I was doing in circuits, if it hadn't been for getting started with something then I dread to imagine what sort of condition I would be in now. Those circuit exercises got me back to dancing, and for that I am eternally grateful. It took time and it has taken three years to get back to where I was in my dance training, but it has been worth all the effort, and my story continues throughout this book.

Kay, an HMSA group leader, wanted to return to running. She describes her experience in the box below.

Running and HMS

'Not with your joints,' I've heard. 'It's bad for you.'
I'm not a doctor or physio, but it is good for:

- Gluteals – these muscles are important stabilisers, generally need strengthening and running uses them. In the bad old days, they didn't recruit in me, but now they do, running is an easy way of exercising them. NB, the treadmill doesn't recruit them. I presume the band pulls the feet back and so the lazy glutes can get away without bothering, my hamstrings get cheesed off, play up, spasm, legs twist even at slow speeds. I don't have any of these problems on terra firma despite physios telling me to only run on a treadmill!

- Thoracics – mine were completely rigid for 8 years or more. Physios told me off and told me to practise rotation, but the only rotation in my spine (apart from my neck and there wasn't much there even!) was in my very loose dislocating SIJs [sacroiliac joints] which led to numb feet, every physio denied possible. I did a lung capacity test and was so bad I had to go back 6 weeks later and do it again. Same result – just abandoned as assumed the patient was lying about not having asthma! Now, 10 years later I'm sure it was due to my rigid thoracics. Some physios even said that was good to protect the vital organs! But no it isn't. Some tried acupuncture but my rigid muscles broke the needles. Then I had botox and denervation to the thoracic spine and discovered the rotation I had been missing, which took an enormous amount of strain off the traumatised SIJs. Also I discovered lateral breathing into the ribcage which enabled me to stop using the accessory breathing muscles in my neck I believe and take a lot of strain off my exhausted fibrotic neck muscles. I followed this up with prolotherapy. So I think the thoracics are an underestimated, underchecked 'silent terrorist' part of the body. They tend to stiffen and it is so important to keep them mobile. If I am unable to maintain this now with exercise, stretching, foam rolling, etc., I shall have more prolotherapy (as other key body parts). It made such an enormous difference! You may not know what you are missing. Running (deep breathing) is the best way I know of to give the thoracics a good loosening.

- Weight-bearing exercise – so important for bone health, especially in us with suspicion of weaker bones.

- Cardiovascular benefits – also important for everyone. Correctly there is much emphasis on core stability but cardiovascular activity is important for us too. This was emphasised to me recently when I got a voluntary job helping at the local Community Cardiac Group's aerobics classes. These are mostly elderly people with cardiac (and other) medical problems and it is important for their CV health that they carefully do CV exercise that many of us with joint problems can't do.

- Motivation – what keeps me doing all the core stability exercises, practising on one leg, proprioception, wobble board exercises, checking my foot pronation etc. What is important for running is also important for HMS. Disciplines such as pacing are familiar concepts in running-world.

- Shoulders – when rigid in the 'zombie years', especially after a day at the office in front of the computer, running did loosen them up nicely.

- Sleep – a good sleep aid. My body knocks me out before I do another few miles. Then I sleep better, wake up more refreshed and sleep is when most healing takes place.

- Endorphins – I'm told I just do it for the endorphins. I'm not sure they kick in at low mileage or intensity, but nevertheless, fresh air, exercise and saying hello to a few fellow runners, ducks and squirrels lifts the mood.

Of course, running isn't for everyone. But if it is your cup of tea, and you used to love it, there is no reason why you shouldn't look into it as part of a well-balanced rounded weekly exercise programme. Of course everything in moderation, and for me it falls into the category, like swimming, bodypump, painting, vacuuming, never on consecutive days, never more than twice a week and not more than once a week unless all is very well.

It isn't the same as walking. I used to be better running than walking, with my right leg giving way frequently walking but never running. For a while the left leg was a problem running. There are subtle differences between running and walking, for example running recruits the glutes a lot more while they are not really required for walking.

If anyone is thinking about running, I strongly recommend the right trainers and orthotics to control any overpronation and as well as any other foot abnormalities and also good core stability and hip stability first. Then to build up very slowly and remember pacing. (Kay, aged 44)

PACING

One of the strongest reasons for me attending a pain management course was so that I could learn to pace activity. Pacing is:

doing small amounts of regular activity that is guided by time rather than pain. People often say they are using pain level as a cue to stop activity. The aim of pacing is to stop doing something before the pain increases. (Daniel 2010, p.134)

Pacing was something I had personally been very bad about in the past, and it is a very familiar pattern for patients with chronic pain to do activity in 'boom and bust' cycles. The following excerpt from my pain management journal written during the course might clarify boom and bust.

Physio V came along next and talked to us about 'Boom and Bust' cycles with activity/inactivity. Basically it follows that a person with chronic pain often waits for a good day in terms of their pain, then does a lot, pushing themselves very hard and then ends up in more pain and rests for a long while. Gradually over time they do less and less and less. V introduced the term 'Pacing' which is definitely going to be a difficult one for me to understand, but a really important term. With pacing it means setting baseline starting points of a certain activity or exercise – for example walking. I might feel comfortable walking for 60 minutes on pain free days, but it is important to do this every day, so we take off at least 20 per cent off that time and some more so that it is an amount I can do realistically without becoming over-exhausted. (Isobel Knight)

Initially everything we did had to be 'paced' and measured – even things like sitting down and standing up.

For me standing is still very difficult. My physiotherapist explained to me why this is.

Hypermobile people have to use an incredible amount of extra energy 'just to be' [because] you are always fighting. You have reduced ligamentous support to give you little idea of where you 'almost' are. You have to keep exploring with each joint, which is even harder when you are just standing. You have to think consciously about it all the time, which is why it takes up so much extra brain power and it becomes so fatiguing, and everyone else does this subconsciously! (Katherine Watkins, personal communication, 22 April 2010)

This helps to explain the obvious fatigue attached to being hypermobile and why pacing something up little by little is very important. When measuring pacing, two measurements are taken of a particular task or exercise. For example, when standing, I would measure my standing tolerance one day and then repeat the measurement the next day, divide by two and minus 20 per cent to get a baseline reading. For instance if I managed to stand for 90 seconds on Monday and 60 seconds on Tuesday, that would be 90 + 60 = 150 seconds.

90 + 60 = 150 seconds
150 ÷ 2 = 75 seconds
75 seconds – 20% [i.e. 15 seconds] = 60 seconds

My baseline starting point for standing would be 60 seconds, which I might then 'pace' up by say 1 second a day.

If I started at 60 seconds on Monday, by the following week I would be on 68 seconds.

Pacing was then applied to all activities, but the principles could be applied to managing things like flare ups, fatigue and pacing-up activities – for example, my return to ballet.

Once I started to get the idea about pacing, it did mean that I started to be able to do things a bit more reliably, whereas in the past I had only done things on good days, and then really paid for it for several days after that.

PSYCHOLOGICAL MANAGEMENT OF PAIN

Much to my surprise, one thing that I found hard when attending the pain management course was not the physical exercises or stretch, but the psychological management of pain. I can now reflect on why this is, and I imagine that my feelings were linked to bereavement and a sense of all the time lost in my life owing to pain and not being able to do the things I enjoyed any more, for example dancing.

The pain management course included sessions on depression and anxiety in relationship to pain. There is growing evidence to suggest a genetic link between HMS and anxiety (Bulbena *et al.* 2004). My pain management course stirred up many feelings that I had either internalised or submerged and bringing them out in the open caused the floodgates to open for me: I remember a number of times feeling angry with the staff who were trying to help me, an anger that is quite out of character for me. Part of the anger was about the fact I was in great denial that I would be suffering chronic pain forever, and I found this extremely difficult to accept at that time.

COGNITIVE BEHAVIOURAL THERAPY

One of the techniques that we were taught was cognitive behavioural therapy (CBT). In essence, CBT is about challenging thought patterns that might not always be useful and replacing negative thoughts, such as catastrophising and imagining the worst, with more realistic ones (Daniel 2010). This is important in relation to pain management and the management of mood swings (see Figure 6.1).

I remember part of the principles of CBT involving taking thoughts to 'thought court', just like a trial by jury. For example, if one of my thoughts was that 'nobody likes me', that might be my own private view, but how realistic is that thought really? If I then spoke to friends and family I expect that they would seriously challenge that thought and then I would need to relinquish the strength of hold on my thought which would then feel less threatening and in turn make me feel better. We are all very good at catastrophising or jumping to conclusions about things – for instance, 'My pain is going to get worse and worse.' The more I believe that thought and the more I am convinced by it, the worse my pain is going to feel regardless of how bad it is in reality, and I am making things even worse by the power of my mind. Once practised, the principles of CBT can help to challenge such thoughts and feelings and (we hope) moderate them and make things a little more realistic. None of this is easy and it needs regular practice. The principles need to be taught by a professional and not just learned from reading the suggestions outlined here.

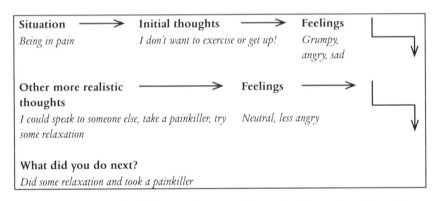

Figure 6.1: An example of the use of CBT and its application to thoughts and feelings in relation to pain

The principles of CBT could be used to manage all manner of moods including ones related to being in pain and difficulties with HMS. One thing that is difficult for me is in snapping back into my knees and locking into my knee hyperextension. I am always being reminded about this by my Pilates teacher, my ballet teacher and, to an extent, my physiotherapist.

Sometimes I feel fed up about it and think I cannot be bothered about it – but see what happens to my thought patterns (Figure 6.2).

CBT can be used for all sorts of situations and to help with strong emotions such as anxiety, depression and anger which are so inextricably linked with HMS and pain. There are two other useful adjuncts to pain and the psychological management of pain – these are relaxation and goal-setting.

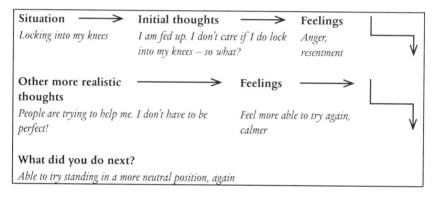

Figure 6.2: An example of the use of CBT and its application to thoughts and feelings in relation to locking into my joints

RELAXATION

Another important aspect to pain management includes 'relaxation techniques'. The worse the pain or fatigue that we experience becomes, the more physically and psychologically 'tense' we become. The more tension increases, the worse the pain and/or fatigue, and it becomes a vicious cycle. Incorporating relaxation techniques into each day is potentially a useful strategy in managing this tension. In fact everyone should do this, not just individuals who are managing pain and other symptoms. There is so much stress in everyday life that some companies invite stress management experts in to work with their staff, but there are basic things that we can all do to help.

Use of breath is an important relaxation technique generally. Have a think about your own breathing patterns next time you are feeling angry, stressed or in pain. You might notice that your breathing rate increases, but the inhalations and exhalations also become more rapid. In relaxation our aim is to slow this process down and decrease the speed of breathing, while maximising intake of nourishing oxygen and removing carbon dioxide. Many somatic (mind–body) practices, for example yoga and Pilates, incorporate breathing into each movement or exercise. Using breath in this way can help with the 'effort' of the movement and so one relaxes into it. Breath can also be useful when stretching as it helps to increase and deepen the stretch that we are trying to achieve. Use of breath is important in relaxation as the aim is to release tension, and make us feel calmer. It is also used as part of meditation practices and so one relaxation that I learned involved counting inhalations up to ten and then starting from one again as a way of retaining focus and concentration. The same could be repeated on counting exhalations instead. Relaxation can also be used as a technique to help with sleep since pain and aching joints and fatigue are all known sleep-robbers.

GOAL-SETTING

Another pain management and HMS strategy involves goal-setting as a way of motivating oneself towards something we want to attain. The SMART principle is useful for goal-setting to ensure that your goals are realistic and achievable:

- **S**pecific
- **M**easurable
- **A**chievable
- **R**ealistic
- **T**ime frame.

Not everybody finds the goal-setting aspects useful and I recall times when I felt it was unhelpful, but it is important to remember that 'Rome wasn't built in a day' and not to be hard on yourself when you are not able to achieve all that you want. HMS is a difficult condition and the instability in the body caused by the general collagenous laxity makes things very changeable. Breaking larger goals down into smaller steps can help when you feel you cannot see right to the end. Remember to keep asking for the support and recognition from others of your hard work and effort. Just 'being' is sometimes difficult in an unstable body, and it is OK to have a bad day!

CONCLUSION

It can be extremely hard coping with a medical condition that causes excessive pain, but doing exercise is a vital part of its management. People with HMS frequently present to physiotherapists and other medical professionals in a deconditioned state and have often reduced activity owing to kinesiophobia (fear of movement). The return to exercise must be done slowly and carefully under medical supervision (initially) and, although strength training might understandably predominate, cardiovascular training and stretching hypermobile areas should not be ignored (Simmonds and Keer 2007, 2008).

Although some examples of exercises have been given in this chapter and in Chapter 7, I have deliberately avoided pictures of different strengthening exercises because everyone has different needs and the physiotherapist or trainer working with you will create your own programme. There is also a danger of people attempting exercises from pictures and it is not my intention that you replicate my programme, although you might encounter similar exercises yourself.

In this chapter we have explored HMS from a pain management point of view, looking at:

- acute pain

- chronic pain

- sensitised sensation and pain amplification

- pain management – analgesia

- management of chronic pain

- attending a residential pain management course

- exercise – stretching

- exercise – circuits

- pacing

- psychological management of pain

- cognitive behavioural therapy

- relaxation

- goal-setting.

Nobody should have to manage alone and in pain and so you should always consult with your own GP for advice and support in terms of pain medication. Chapter 9 discusses the psychological implications of HMS and Chapter 11 goes into further detail in ways in which to manage HMS.

CHAPTER 7

Other Related Physical Conditions and HMS

HMS can seem to be just about joints and being hypermobile, but many other symptoms and medical conditions are now being shown to be linked to HMS. The physical conditions are dealt with in this chapter, while anxiety and other psychological links are discussed in Chapter 9. The effects of menstruation and hormonally related conditions (including pregnancy) are described in Chapter 8.

In Chapter 2 the diversity of HMS was illustrated with body systemic links (e.g. digestive system) to a range of different health conditions. This chapter goes into more detail about some of the most commonly reported conditions, but it cannot cover all syndrome-related conditions, so if one of your symptoms is not mentioned here, it might have been acknowledged in Chapter 2. New links are currently being made with HMS and other conditions. Please discuss it with your own doctor, who might be able to enlighten you further.

Research is collectively showing a link with HMS and conditions related to dysautonomia and malfunctioning of the autonomic nervous system. The ANS is responsible for functions which we would normally take for granted and for the body to deal with subconsciously (hence being called autonomic) such as heart rate, temperature and bowel function. When aspects of the ANS fail to work as well as they should, the outcome can include problems with the bowel, including nausea and diarrhoea, and problems with the heart rate, including dizziness and tachycardia (fast heart rate). These conditions are commonly found in patients with HMS and EDS quite possibly owing to the presence of abnormally elastic connective tissue and loss of supporting connective tissues in vascular tissues (Kanjwal *et al.* 2009). It is also not surprising that some people with postural orthostatic tachycardia syndrome are frequently misdiagnosed, and are instead diagnosed with anxiety or panic disorders, which are also linked with HMS (Bulbena *et al.* 2004). ANS dysfunction with conditions such as chronic fatigue syndrome and fibromyalgia also shares symptomatic links with HMS (Nijs 2005). Research into ANS dysfunction and connective tissue disorders continues.

POSTURAL ORTHOSTATIC TACHYCARDIA SYNDROME

One minute I am crouching to look at books at the bottom row of the library; the next minute I am holding on to the walls and shelves of the library for dear life to stop myself blacking out... Sometimes when I get out of bed, I see lots of stars and the room spins... After I have danced I have to get my head down quickly, lest I should faint... I am just watching the TV (nothing scary!) and my heart rate accelerates from normal to 100 miles an hour. Randomly! (Isobel Knight)

Postural orthostatic tachycardia syndrome is caused by disturbances to the ANS. Patients with POTS might complain of symptoms such as tachycardia (palpitations), fatigue, lightheadedness, exercise intolerance, nausea, headache, mental clouding or brain-fog and syncope (fainting). It is a condition that affects females to males in a ratio of four to one, and is related to other autoimmune conditions such as irritable bowel syndrome and HMS. The most striking physical feature of POTS is a severe (and sometimes delayed) tachycardia that develops on standing from lying down (Raj 2006).

The blood volume is low in many POTS patients and POTS can be measured by use of a laboratory tilt test which measures the heart rate and blood pressure of a patient on the horizontal and vertical plane, the variance in blood pressure and rise in heart rate indicating presence of POTS. If you suspect that you have POTS, your doctor will advise you appropriately on the management of this condition. Medication might be suggested such as the use of Duloxetine, an SSRI which has been shown to alter the autonomic tone (Kanjwal et al. 2009).

No medicines are officially approved by the US Food and Drug Administration for the treatment of POTS. Patients should avoid factors that might exacerbate POTS such as extreme heat and dehydration. Further management strategies include exercising to reverse deconditioning, but the return to exercise must be slowly paced since essentially overly rigorous exercise too soon may worsen symptoms and initially prolong fatigue (Raj 2006). Research into POTS in relation to HMS and other connective tissue and ANS-related disorders continues.

GASTROINTESTINAL DISORDERS

Hannah (aged 11) has diabolical symptoms. Her gut problem goes on all day long and she cannot go to school. She feels really sick all day long, and full, and terrible. It is like a nightmare. She is too ill for school and gets pain in her ankle and knee all the time. It has just been so depressing. HMS is a very sad condition. No one understands it. (Hannah's mother)

Research is now beginning to show links between HMS and functional gastrointestinal disorders (FGIDs) such as irritable bowel disorder and heartburn. Other symptoms include abdominal bloating, constipation and diarrhoea. Nausea and vomiting have also been reported (Aziz ND). Research started when it became clear that increasing numbers of HMS patients reported having gastrointestinal symptoms on their visits, notably to Professor Grahame and Dr Hakim's London clinics. HMS patients were two times more likely to have Crohn's disease in the Greek Caucasian population, while there was no difference in ulcerative colitis compared to the healthy control group (Vounotrypidis et al. 2009).

An unknown cause for gastrointestinal symptoms is significantly more frequent in people with joint hypermobility than those without. In one study, 63 of 129 patients (49%) were hypermobile. Of a further 25 patients, 17 (68%) were diagnosed with HMS and experienced the following symptoms: abdominal pain (81%), bloating (57%), nausea (57%), reflux symptoms (48%), vomiting (43%), constipation (38%) and diarrhoea (14%) (Zarate *et al.* 2009). The study concluded that further research is required in linking connective tissue to unexplained gastrointestinal symptoms. The sluggish gut symptoms might relate to the general tissue laxity and increased elasticity found in the tissue of hypermobile people. This might then explain why the gut behaves in a less efficient way, because of the flexibility of the tissues. Further research continues in all areas, and it is hoped that the future includes newer treatments and pharmaceutical interest (Aziz ND).

Management of pan-gastrointestinal symptoms and IBS involves looking at diet as well as the use of medication to help with some of the symptoms. Smoking, alcohol, caffeine and stress are all likely to contribute to symptoms as will potentially eating very spicy foods – especially to those who suffer from heartburn and upper gastrointestinal symptoms such as indigestion and reflux. Chewing food more carefully makes good common sense, but many HMS patients have problems with their jaws and so chewing food is sometimes difficult and fatiguing. Chewing gum should be avoided. The type of medication required will depend on the nature of the symptoms. For example, taking an antacid for indigestion might help that symptom, while another type of medication might be required to relax the painful spasms in the intestines and lower gut which accompany the condition. Medication might also help with the problems arising from alternating diarrhoea and constipation which sufferers of IBS will be only too aware of. At an academic London Hypermobility meeting, some experts recommended looking at general toilet behaviour – for example, in ensuring that one uses the bathroom as soon as one has a desire to go rather than waiting for a more convenient time. Posture on the toilet was also remarked on because piles and anal polyps are commonly related symptoms in people who regularly suffer from constipation. Psychology might have a role and this might be important in retraining sluggish bowels and an urge to use the bathroom (Zarate *et al.* 2009).

ASTHMA

One day I had an audibly wheezy chest and my GP prescribed steroid tablets and increasingly stronger inhalers, but my 'peak flow', which measures lung capacity on exhalation, was not showing particularly low – my average reading seemed to be 350 (my usual reading is 500). After a few days of increasing steroid intakes and no major changes to my peak flow, but no changes to my wheezy chest, my GP put me on a nebuliser, measured my peak flow again, which had decreased, and then gave me a second nebuliser treatment. There was no change or improvement. She then decided to put me on a course of antibiotics and suggested I attended A&E if there were no further improvements. She was contemplating sending me there directly, but we decided to see if the antibiotics worked. My GP said she was quite puzzled by my lack of response to the nebulisers and even started to wonder if I was allergic to one of the drugs administered. The next morning I felt slightly worse again and so went to A&E, as advised. The A&E doctors were equally baffled. They could hear my very audibly wheezy chest and yet as before my peak flow wasn't disastrous. I mentioned that I had HMS, but they failed to make a connection between that and asthma. They questioned whether I was indeed experiencing asthma and discharged me without taking any further action. Two days later I returned to my GP and she sent me for a chest X-ray, which was normal. I mentioned to my GP an article I had found on asthma and airway collapse in heritable disorders of connective tissue (Morgan *et al.* 2007). A later informal discussion with my rheumatologist confirmed that the unusual peak flow and my slightly strange response to medication did seem related to the HMS and an increased lung capacity owing to systemic collagen laxity.

Research does indeed show that 'increased lung volumes, impaired gas transfer, increased lung compliance and an increased tendency of the airways to collapse...genes contributing to asthma and either HMS or EDS may be in linkage' (Morgan *et al.* 2007, p.1327). It seems that the stretchy collagens found in HMS patients means that their lung capacity is potentially greater. Ongoing monitoring of asthma in these patients, peak flow monitoring and conventional inhaled therapy treatment are recommended.

SKIN – HEALING, SCARRING, STRETCH MARKS AND BRUISING

I have such soft and velvety skin that I can only wash most of my skin using baby lotion and witch hazel. Soap and water are too abrasive for most of my body. (Jenny, aged 64)

Faulty collagens mean that the skin does not always heal and might well have a more fragile and 'papery' texture, or seem almost 'rubbery' with the stretchy collagen fibres (Russek 1999; Simpson 2006). The skin is often much more easily damaged and needs to be more carefully handled – for example by bodywork practitioners such as physiotherapists and other complementary health practitioners.

FIBROMYALGIA AND FATIGUE

Saturday, 25 September 2010

The cat's hourly rate has increased. He is definitely working overtime because I am literally grounded. I spent most of Saturday afternoon in and out of bed. I got up to try and eat and then achieve something. I am in tip to toe pain with very nasty nodules. I feel like I have the flu. My cold has come back again and skin wounds are not healing. This morning I had to go and feed my neighbour's cat. I did so and had to go back to bed. The effort was just too much. (Isobel Knight)

Since both fibromyalgia and HMS are common in the general population, it is not surprising to find both fibromyalgia and HMS occurring in any one individual by chance. Patients with fibromyalgia describe chronic widespread pain and other symptoms, notably sleep disturbance and fatigue, which are symptoms often shared by HMS patients. In fibromyalgia, the muscles are often tight due to a lack of relaxation. It is as if they cannot switch the muscles off, and this has also been my personal experience of treating patients with fibromyalgia using the Bowen technique. The sleep disturbance in fibromyalgic patients suggests that they do not show a normal decreased sympathetic nervous system (fight or flight) between 2am and 5am compared to normal controls. It seems they have a very fragmented deep sleep and this very much tallies with HMS patients (Rahman and Holman 2010).

There is certainly a relationship between fibromyalgia, HMS and autonomic dysfunction – for example the symptoms of POTS and pan-gastrointestinal disorders, both described in this chapter. It is the development of faults within the ANS, 'dysautonomia', which is the strongest connection between HMS and fibromyalgia (Rahman and Holman 2010).

> Clinical autonomic dysfunctions abound, including abnormal thermoregulation, palpitations, excessive gastric acidity and irritable bowel syndrome, irritable bladder, restless legs syndrome, bruxism and sleep disturbance... Heightened arousal, vigilance and fear also influence the intensity of anxiety, post traumatic stress disorder (PTSD)... HMS and fibromyalgia appear to predispose to greater autonomic responsiveness to appropriate sympathetic arousals: stress, fear etc... In turn, subjects possibly react with greater vigor and duration; repetitive painful stimuli likely heighten the autonomic response over time. (Rahman and Holman 2010, pp.64–65)

The overlap with fibromyalgia and HMS – this is an interesting question. They don't diagnose HMS in the USA. Rheumatologists are aware of its existence, but see it as a chronic pain problem and many would fit in to the concept of fibromyalgia. There is clearly a lot of overlap as it has not been adequately researched; certainly for HMS patients who have chronic pain, some will have the tender points linked to fibromyalgia, but the diagnostic criteria for fibromyalgia might be changing. There is an overlap and many fibromyalgia patients are hypermobile and many HMS patients have chronic pain with tender points. It has to be more coincidence in the end. (Professor Rodney Grahame, personal communication, 20 October 2010)

The shared symptoms with the ANS (e.g. dizziness, palpitations) in patients with HMS and fibromyalgia make this a starting point for further research into the shared 'pathophysiology' between these two conditions.

FLAT FEET

Figure 7.1 depicts someone with flat feet.

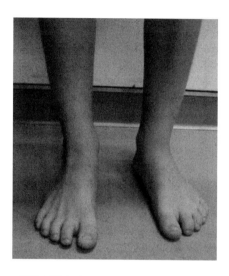

Figure 7.1: 'Flat feet' arch collapse owing to tissue laxity – there is some eversion of the right foot, and pronation of the left

The medial arch is supported by ligaments and muscles and so it is not a constructive mortice as a bony arch, therefore if you have got a connective tissue problem like HMS, with lax collagen, then those ligaments and muscle and fascia supporting the longitudinal arch will flatten under gravity with the weight of the body. It is just the tissues, stretchy and lax, collapse under the weight of the body, which is why they 'self-correct' when not supported by weight. The other aspect controlling the arch is the subtalar joint which has got some bony support, but people will pronate again because of weight-bearing on the soft tissues, but if they have more eversion, they will appear to be less flat-footed. (Dr Jane Simmonds, personal communication, 14 August 2010)

Having flat feet, fallen arches or excessive pronation (ankles rolling in) seem to be synonymous with HMS, although the reasons underlying this seem to be poorly understood. One reason for flat feet might be linked to a faulty 'locking and unlocking mechanism' in the feet of HMS patients. In 'normal' feet, there exists a subtle locking and unlocking mechanism which allows the foot to cope with uneven ground and act as a lever in walking, and this mechanism might be slightly impaired in HMS patients (Redmond ND). An unstable ankle joint could contribute to flat feet and also skin fragility. Some HMS patients tend to have a scoliosis (curvature of the spine) which can lead to unequal leg length and 'angular rotation of the feet on walking' (Bird 2007b, p.16). Such patients should receive podiatric attention and orthotic appliances might be beneficial.

People with HMS should take care to consider their footwear, ensuring that it provides adequate support. Court-style shoes, which are tight at the heel, are unsuitable; trainers are recommended because the materials can be breathable, they have laces that support and also shock-absorbing soles. Physical therapy exercises to strengthen the feet would be beneficial and exercises that work to strengthen joint proprioception and the way in which the HMS person perceives their sense of balance and joint position. Experts advocate the need for foot-care and adequate management and treatment of conditions such as bunions and hammer toes, and the need for surgical management, if this is required (Redmond ND; Tinkle 2008).

MUSCLE CRAMPING AND SPASMING

Tuesday, 2 February 2010

Things have been slightly difficult since I had a physiotherapy session which produced a big reaction and therefore major changes in me. At the moment I am still having problems with spasms which I am presently calling 'Eenie Meenie Miney Moe'. Meenie is the big one from my spine that kicks off when I am sitting on certain seats – mostly bus or train seats. He also kicks off when I am lying flat or doing certain spinal extension work. Eenie is a cute little kick into my left side, Miney is my abdominal spasm and Moe is a diaphragmatic one. I don't get Moe too often. Anyway – I decided lately that the best way to cope with them was to befriend them, so I (sort of) have. The thing I am finding difficult is that it looks like I am having some sort of minor fit or seizure and makes me a feel a bit of a freak when it happens in public or in Pilates. Last week at almost the end of Pilates I had a big attack of Meenie, but I cried too because I was tired of what precisely was going on. There is never any pain attached to Meenie, but perhaps an emotional response. I am now taking occasional Baclofan for Meenie because he also objects to bedtime and me lying flat. Eenie also enjoys night-time for fun and kicks. (Isobel Knight)

A visit to my local A&E Department ended inconclusively at the helm of another HMS-related symptom. Although I had been suffering regular episodes of muscle spasms as described above, one day I was in a meeting at work. I was feeling well. I was not caffeinated, stressed or anxious. During the middle of the meeting, I felt a sudden surge of heat up to my brain followed by a change in pulse rate and temperature and accompanied by immediate brain-fogging and feeling as though I had been put on 'pause'. I tried to continue the rest of the meeting as calmly as possible, but developed a sudden headache and feeling of 'pressure' in my head. I didn't know what was happening to me, but it was extremely unpleasant. I managed to complete my meeting and then had to go into another one almost straight away. I managed to conduct the second meeting in a matter of minutes and alluded to feeling unwell. I then managed to get back to the clinic rooms at work: working in the health department has its advantages. I had already put some Bowen moves into my body which would normally have taken it out of shock, but on this occasion lying down and trying to rest seemed to agitate things further. Several other things happened simultaneously. I began to have very large and systemic muscle spasms that again stemmed from my spine, and was twitching away (see the above account), and I felt extremely cold and was shivering (it was a very muggy July day) and became very clammy. Not feeling very comfortable about things, I asked one of my colleagues to sit with me and requested them to ask for two of the Pilates staff who knew about my muscle spasms and my condition in general.

The Pilates staff arrived and couldn't believe what they were seeing. I said that I would feel more comfortable in moving gently so I walked to the Pilates studio, which was fortunately empty given that it was lunchtime. I felt the need to lie with my head on a semi-inflated ball (known as an over-ball) and one instructor placed my legs over a foam triangle. It was hopeless in this position and I was arching all over the place right the way through my whole spine. It looked like I was having a major seizure. Sitting up seemed to improve things a bit, but the spasms and muscular 'twitches' continued. After a further hour with nothing stopping them and a very nasty headache, my colleagues felt that I should be checked out in hospital. I was generally resistant to the idea because I didn't think that they would be able to do anything. However, my colleagues later disclosed they had anxieties about me because of the severe headaches and wanted to ensure that nothing more sinister was going on (stroke).

I finally started to warm up in the car. When we arrived at A&E it was apparent that there was going to be a long wait. I was eventually given a thorough examination and had an ECG and full blood and infection counts done, which were all normal. I was given a drip of fluids and salts and my urine was tested, which revealed the beginnings of a possible infection, but nothing remarkable. Blood pressure was apparently normal, including pressure taken on lying down and standing. There was nothing in my chemistry that could apparently account for these strange events, which were behaving in the manner of POTS. The doctors could not believe the spasms and had no idea what was causing them and why they were continuing so relentlessly. I had to convince them this was not a panic attack! They discharged me because this was A&E and they had achieved their role in eliminating anything life-threatening or sinister. They suggested plenty of rest, painkillers and fluids, and no work next day. They also suggested that my GP should refer me to be reviewed by my rheumatologist sooner rather than later to investigate the cause of the muscle spasms. This was another example of peculiar HMS-related symptoms, where the A&E doctors were unable to determine the cause and solution of muscle spasms and waves of twitches. I had suspected that it would be a waste of time in attending A&E but needed to appease my work colleagues of nothing more serious going on. Also this had been the first time that I had experienced an episode of muscle spasms triggered by a vascular incident and independent of physiotherapy, Bowen or Pilates.

The muscle spasms and twitches continued for almost 12 hours after the original trigger. The spasms had a resultant effect on my bowels and bladder and over the next few days my abdominal muscles were sore beyond belief, coupled with wider spread pain into my arms and into my hip flexors and adductor (inner thigh) leg muscles. I didn't tell many people about this episode in the end because I felt so drained with the experience and yet another unfathomable HMS symptom. Attempting to explain some of the mysteries of this condition can become endlessly tiring not least because people don't understand what is happening. I am lucky in that my Pilates instructors (incidentally friends and colleagues) are well aware of my HMS and also had witnessed me having spasm attacks before. I wouldn't like to have to attempt to explain this to non-medical friends, or further alarm my family. Some things are better left unsaid. When I got home I realised I had my HMSA membership card, which provides a brief explanation of HMS. Next time I end up in A&E I will show them that. In the mean time I am awaiting a follow-up rheumatology appointment and future investigation into the cause of the spasms. Judging by other HMSA online (and moderated) forum users' experiences, even if I am sent for neurological investigation, it may still not unearth the cause of my muscle spasms; it may be left to further medical research and knowledge pooling to explain their occurrence.

Myocolonus means spasm of muscle and JHS people do get it. Joints can be so loose (probably collagen structure) so spasm is a protective mechanism. Or a spasm may be a musculoskeletal phenomenon that is linked to those who have hypermobility as a result of neurological tone – for example abnormal proprioception group [all conjecture and Professor Bird's suspicion]. Some of the abnormalities of the spine are linked to muscle spasms, just as some neurological diseases such as MS.

Management – careful history needed; all over body is a different ball park to joints that are often the most hypermobile.

Autonomic neuropathy – POTS might link to blood pressure/ pulse rate might link with the muscular control. (Professor Howard Bird, personal communication, 29 April 2010)

If there are muscle spasms, they are related to pain – spasms, protective spasm or a psychological protective spasm because of that. Sometimes people get twitching and this can be because of hypersensitivity of the nervous system because they have that in addition to their connective tissue disorder, associated with, or because you can get, perturbation of the muscle because of fatigue, or a nutritional problem to the muscle, so you might get some fatigue element and perturbation there. The spasms are not a condition of the nervous system and some people might have delayed motor control, but not everyone has this and HMS is a connective tissue disorder, not a neurological disorder. (Dr Jane Simmonds, personal communication, 14 August 2010)

OSTEOPOROSIS AND OSTEOPENIA

There is an increased risk of bone fragility, fracture and future osteoporosis in patients with HMS (Bird 2007b). The increased risk of fracture might be owing to regular trauma via falls, dislocations and other HMS-related incidents. The increased incidence of brittle bones or osteoporosis in HMS patients might be related to the general connective tissue and collagenous disorder; however, this is speculative, rather than proven.

HMS increases the risk for low bone mass or osteopenia; pre-menopausal women with joint hypermobility have lower bone mineral density when compared to control groups, and hypermobility increases the risk for low bone mass (Gulbahar et al. 2006). People with osteopenia are certainly at greater risk of later developing osteoporosis, but there are things that might combat this development, such as ensuring the diet has sufficient quantities of Vitamin D and calcium. Bones need 'stress' to lay down more bone, so weight-bearing exercise is useful to promote bone growth. In HMS patients who are very inactive, it might be easier to see why they are potentially more prone to osteopenia. This is therefore another good reason to exercise, if you can.

Osteopenia and osteoporosis are investigated with 'DEXA' scans, which measure bone density in the lumbar spine and pelvis (DEXA means dual energy X-ray absorptiometry). Your physician would advise if you needed to be monitored for osteopenia, which is another symptom related to HMS. Other related reasons for osteopenia include amenorrhoea or irregular menstruation. Bone repair is dependent on oestrogen since the hormone prevents bone loss (Manore and Thompson 2000). Absence of menstruation is caused when a woman's weight and energy levels drop below a level to sustain the menstrual cycle. Osteoporosis is the resultant loss of bone density, through amenorrhoea, which greatly increases the risk of stress fractures. Dancers are particularly at risk, and given that there is such a high prevalence of hypermobility within the dance world, the importance of bone health, adequate diet and appropriate (contraceptive) medication to regulate menses must be emphasised in this group. Dancers therefore need educating to understand the importance of regular menstruation in terms of bone health, the lack of which could destroy their career (Chartrand and Chatfield 2005; Frusztajer *et al.* 1990).

OSTEOARTHRITIS

There is still limited information on this. The Chingford epidemiological study where 1000 women were surveyed every year for 10–15, possibly 20, years for osteoarthritis and osteoporosis showed that people who had traces of HM or HMS were better placed in terms of osteoarthritis and osteoporosis and it was regarded as a fitness factor. There may be a population of hypermobile people who actually benefit from it as they have less osteoarthritis than other people. This is a conundrum – an open question as we don't know the answer! (Professor Rodney Grahame, personal communication, 20 October 2010)

Research is conflicting as to whether there is an increased risk of premature osteoarthritis (PO) of the temporomandibular joint (TMJ, or jaw) and of the knee and hand in HMS patients. There are insufficient data to say whether there is increased risk in the general population, but there is evidence of increased risk in those who work hypermobile joints hard, such as dancers. Professor Grahame examined the onset of osteoarthritis and saw 75 dancers. Those aged 29 and below were classed as young dancers, and those over 30 as older dancers: 89 per cent of the young dancers and 79 per cent of the older ones satisfied HMS criteria.

Some problems included:

- non-inflammatory joint pain

- arthralgia

- low back pain.

In young dancers, the overriding complaints were soft-tissue injuries. In older dancers, the overriding problems were hip problems and osteoarthritis (Grahame 2009c).

In terms of knee osteoarthritis, the onset of osteoarthritis is as much to do with one's genetic fate as with hypermobility. Prehabilitation in advance of surgery is recommended, so that the surrounding tissues in the hypermobile patient are strengthened as much as possible which would also speed recovery (knowing that the skin and soft-tissue healing time in hypermobiles is often slower) (Haddad and Dhawan 2010).

It is probable that hypermobility hastens or increases the likelihood of a person getting osteoarthritis, particularly in dancers (Grahame 2009a). People with HMS should improve their strength and control and avoid overuse of the joint to minimise the increased risk of osteoarthritis owing to their hypermobility; however, the genetic risk of osteoarthritis remains the same as it would irrespective of hypermobility (Butler 2010).

Is hypermobility advantageous as you get older?

I think it is starting to tip into the negative because when I was younger I mean I suppose I could use particularly my arms and shoulders, I could be flexible and stuff, but I remember the physiotherapists who were horrified how I lifted my rucksack onto my right arm and shoulder – so I had proper lessons on how to do it. They were really good to me because they always picked me up when I crashed. So I made use of my flexibility and I am stiffening up. I am stiffening up and don't think my fingers aren't nearly as flexible as they used to be – my thumbs certainly aren't and I have wear and tear in the joints from all the therapy work I used to do. (Grace, aged 65)

PROLAPSES

People with HMS are more prone to abdominal, rectal and uterine prolapses (and hernias) owing to weakness of the connective tissues and muscular-supporting structures and general tissue laxity (Tinkle 2008). Women with joint hypermobility have a significantly higher prevalence of genital prolapse compared to women with normal mobility, and ageing, hormones, pregnancy and trauma also contribute to prolapses (Norton *et al.* 1995). Women with HMS and pelvic organ prolapse could be more likely to sustain heavy post-operative bleeding during surgery to correct prolapse, although it is unclear why this is the case. Treatment to minimise blood loss and bleeding is recommended (Kinsler *et al.* 2008).

WEAKENED BLADDER

Weakened collagen and tissue laxity mean that the bladder can be affected in some people with HMS (see the interview with Natasha on p.67 for her experience of this). Treatment options include working on improving the muscular support of the pelvic floor, medication such as Duloxetine, and using a pessary, a plastic device which supports the bladder (or uterus). In more serious cases corrective surgery might also be required (Norton *et al.* 1995; Tinkle 2008).

VARICOSE VEINS

I have varicose veins – have had them since I was a teenager. I also have extremely poor circulation, which possibly goes with the varicose veins. If my wrists or ankles are not warm, I have had it. It wasn't until I started to do alternative therapies that I had an idea about how that affects you (energetic work). You still have to live though and get on with it. Then there is all the other things like bladder – I have always had a weak bladder. Pelvic floor not brilliant! (Grace, aged 65)

People with HMS might be more prone to having varicose veins owing to their tissue laxity (Grahame 2010). It is another diagnostic sign of weakened tissues and forms part of the Brighton criteria.

VISITING THE DENTIST AND TMJ PROBLEMS

What follows is my experience of visiting the dentist.

When I open my mouth it is not in a straight line, or smooth movement at all. My TMJ gets stuck. The joint is painful and in me is not at all hypermobile, but it is excessively clicky and keeping it open wide – for example for the dentist – is extremely difficult. My dentist is very good to me and lets me take regular breaks when I need to. Fortunately I only have one filling so far and my problems are more structural rather than related to decay. I have an orthodontic splint which I wear at night which gives my TMJ a rest and in particular the soft tissues which are working so very hard. This has been extremely successful. (Isobel Knight)

There is a link between hypermobility and problems with the TMJ with a ratio of five to one for women; the peak age for symptoms is 15–30 years old and over 40 for degenerative joint disease (Bryden 2010; Dijkstra, Kropmans and Stregenga 2002). Factors indicative of TMJ symptoms include orofacial pain, joint sounds and looking at the range of movement in opening the jaw. Physiotherapy might help with TMJ symptoms including careful assessment of the cervical spine. A dental practitioner with an expertise in TMJ dysfunction is invaluable, for example by providing corrective splinting (Bryden 2010).

The management of TMJ dysfunction includes reducing an initial inflammation, for example by use of gentle heat, ice or ultrasound. It is recommended that excessive gum chewing is avoided and that patients opt for a more soft-food diet. Dental splinting might be helpful and assist with other aspects such as bruxism or grinding the teeth. Physiotherapy exercises might also be beneficial. When visiting the dentist, breaks will be necessary to give the TMJ a rest (Bryden 2010).

CONCLUSION

In this chapter we have looked at a range of conditions related to having HMS. Some of these closely link in with dysfunction of the ANS such as POTS and IBS. Others are related to faulty collagens and excessive tissue laxity such as asthma, flat feet, varicose veins, weak bladder and prolapses.

Other conditions such as fibromyalgia and problems with muscle spasms and fatigue also relate to having chronic pain, resultant of continuous injury and soft-tissue trauma at the helm of tissue laxity.

Research continues into all areas and it is likely that as the medical professionals collaborate more symptoms and medical conditions will also be related to HMS. Professor Rodney Grahame's hopes for the future are recorded on p.215. Chapter 9 looks at the psychological conditions related to HMS and how to obtain psychological and social support for HMS.

CHAPTER 8

Menstruation, Pregnancy, Childbirth and the Menopause and HMS

Although joint laxity decreases after puberty, the influence of hormones once menstruation commences in females can have a profound effect on their symptoms and the way in which the joint laxity behaves.

The hormones responsible for the menstrual cycle in females include oestrogen and progesterone. The balance between these two hormones which control the menstrual cycle fluctuates throughout the menstrual cycle. These two hormones are absent prior to menarche (first menstrual period) and decline after the menopause (Bird 2007a). The functions of oestrogen include promoting the calcification of bone, female fat distribution and promoting female hair distribution. The functions of progesterone include supporting the growth of the lining of the uterus and supporting the placenta during pregnancy (Hamilton-Fairley 2004). It is normally the hormone progesterone which is responsible for the increase in symptoms in relation to joint laxity, particularly in those patients who have a higher degree of collagen-type hypermobility (Bird 2007a, 2007b; Knight and Bird 2010).

> Although oestrogen tends to stabilise collagen, progesterones loosen it. Many hypermobile patients, although not all, noticed a worsening of symptoms, more pain in the joints, clumsiness or a great tendency to dislocate in the five days leading up to menstruation and in the few days after menstruation. This is exactly the time when the progesterone compounds far exceed the stabilising oestrogen compounds. (Bird 2007a, p.10)

For women experiencing irregular menstruation, this can make joint symptoms worse for longer because progesterone concentrations remain higher for longer. Irregular periods can mask other gynaecological conditions such as ovarian cysts or endometriosis. The joint deterioration, symptoms and pain alone can suggest these problems before they are more formally diagnosed by a gynaecologist (Bird 2007a, 2007b).

ENDOMETRIOSIS

Endometriosis is a condition in which the endometrium (the lining of the uterus) escapes into the surrounding pelvis and elsewhere (Henderson and Wood 2000). It is a condition that is so far poorly understood. The shed endometrium causes pain and inflammation as the cells attach themselves to other parts of the pelvis and grow in response to the menstrual cycle. Endometriosis can be found in any area of the pelvis including the bladder and bowels. It can also be found (rarely) in the lungs, kidney and diaphragm (Hamilton-Fairley 2004). In a study of 41 adult women with Ehlers-Danlos syndrome, 27 per cent had endometriosis, thus showing prevalence for the condition in the hypermobile population (McIntosh *et al.* 1995).

Symptoms of endometriosis include the following (Mears 1996):

- period pain (dysmenorrhoea)

- painful intercourse (dyspareunia)

- painful ovulation

- infertility

- painful urination

- painful bowel movements

- back pain

- digestive complaints

- fatigue

- depression

- psychological – poor memory and concentration.

Some of the symptoms have a very large cross-over with the symptoms experienced in relation to HMS – in fact when I came to write this section of the book I reviewed some previous research I had conducted into endometriosis, and I found many similarities. This could explain why my diagnosis with HMS has been slow and some of the symptoms masked by other symptoms I have had in relation to having endometriosis. Until I was diagnosed with HMS I did not know that the hormonal influence might exacerbate my symptoms and so undeniably endometriosis has had an effect on my HMS and vice versa. The fact I felt more hypermobile leading up to menstruation, and the fact my back pain and fatigue increased and my injury risk also seemed to increase around my menstrual period, are entirely related to higher progesterone rates which impacted substantially on my HMS symptoms. The implications for the way in which progesterone can affect HMS women is therefore critical to take into account when doctors consider contraceptive and other hormonal treatments.

HORMONAL TREATMENTS AND HMS – CONTRACEPTIVE PILL

Hormones had an impact. In the past I was put on high-dose progesterone pills which made me feel much worse – but it was not until now I could see the impact of this. Professor G diagnosed me and suggested various ways forwards to my GP. (Sara, aged 34)

HMS women who have increased symptoms around their menstrual cycle should certainly check their contraceptive medication with their rheumatologist, gynaecologist or GP to determine whether they are taking a progesterone-only contraceptive pil. It might be that changing the contraceptive pill to a more oestrogen-dominant pill can improve their symptoms and minimise the difficulties that progesterone seems to cause in increasing tissue laxity, pain, dislocations and other symptoms. However, it is up to the GP, rheumatologist or gynaecologist to advise since there might be good reasons for their initial selection of drug. Sometimes an increased oestrogen contraceptive is unwise as there is some potential for an increased risk of breast cancer or thrombosis (Bird 2007a, p.11). However, there are times when a change of contraception would be beneficial if most symptoms are improved.

OTHER HORMONAL MEDICATION

I was given a progesterone implant (Prostap) as one variation of treatment for my endometriosis. All my joint aches and pains seemed to flare significantly, which tallies to the response that other women might have from high-dose progesterone contraceptive pills. Progesterones often tend to exacerbate symptoms and lead to a deterioration in pain and joint laxity (Bird 2004, 2010). Needless to say I requested to come off this medication. A similar incident arose from trying the Mirena coil, which is another progesterone-based medication, the drug being released in small doses from a coil in the uterus. I had a coil inserted following surgical removal of endometriosis. Within weeks following surgery I was in excruciating pain everywhere. Apparently once the nurse removed the coil, which was falling out of place anyway, the relief could be seen almost instantly on my face. These are my personal experiences of such medication, and are based on a secondary condition, endometriosis. Other women might find they work for them. However, since both these drugs are progesterone based, it would make sense for a woman who has HMS and notices an increase in symptoms to mention this to her GP and for alternatives to be suggested.

One aspect of treatment for endometriosis can involve the temporary cessation of the menstrual cycle by means of a monthly hormone injection called Zoladex™, which works by suppressing the hormones that initiate the menstrual cycle, thus creating a temporary and reversible menopause. Hormone replacement therapy (HRT) is administered as add-back therapy since otherwise there are immediate menopausal symptoms that can be difficult for some women to endure such as vaginal dryness and hot flushes. HRT is administered with enough oestrogen so as not to initiate a menstrual cycle, but to prevent too much detrimental bone loss, as that is a problem with this course of treatment. Because my endometriosis is quite severe with symptoms almost certainly enhanced by my HMS and a sensitised nervous system, this treatment has been a lifeline for me. I was regularly being admitted to hospital because my menstrual pain and symptoms were so severe. This treatment means I am in much less pain, but there is a price to pay: because I have been on HRT several times over the years, my bones are now in osteopenia and my bone density is low, leaving me at increased risk of overt osteoporosis in later life. However, I think this is an example of when benefit has outweighed risk. I have been able to live a 'normal' life for the most part, and even though many people cannot tolerate the side effects of Zoladex very well, for me it has been worth it. Every person is different and, if you require hormone medication for endometriosis, contraceptive measure in general or medication for conditions such as polycystic ovarian syndrome (PCOS), a condition which is caused by increased testosterone levels and can cause irregular periods, weight gain and increased facial and body hair (Hamilton-Fairley 2004), your GP, rheumatologist or a gynaecologist will best advise you.

IRREGULAR MENSTRUATION

Absence of menstruation or amenorrhoea is caused when a woman's weight and energy levels drop below a level to sustain the menstrual cycle. Amenorrhoea would certainly need to be eliminated if a woman wishes to conceive. There is currently no research evidence to suggest that women with HMS take any longer than non-HMS women to conceive, but any menstrual or hormonal irregularities would need to be investigated and problems eliminated.

PREGNANCY

Symptoms will get worse during pregnancy and I warn them of that. Most are happy because they are pregnant. I advise them about drugs and medication during pregnancy – for example what to reduce and safety of the foetus. Most want to know if they have risk of death during childbirth and if so early elective Caesarean Section is sometimes advised. The severe types of EDS can occasionally result in death from uterine bleeding and in HMS there is a risk of premature rupture of membranes and rapid delivery. (Professor Howard Bird, personal communication, 29 April 2010)

Just as for non-HMS women, pregnancy can go either way for HMS women. Some will feel better than they do normally, while others will feel much worse. This might be partly related to how they respond to the hormonal conditions of pregnancy, in particular an increase in relaxin, a hormone which relaxes and softens the tissues to prepare the body for labour. During pregnancy there is an 800 per cent rise in uterine collagen content which is reversed after the birth. There is a significant association of hypermobility in low back and pelvic pain during pregnancy, with an overall prevalence of 72 per cent of women being affected. High levels of the hormone relaxin are partially responsible for the most clinically incapacitated. There also reports of increased sacroiliac joint pain and pubic symphysis dysfunction in hypermobile women. The management of pregnancy-related joint pain is similar for HMS women in that support garments such as a prenatal cradle are worn (Grahame and Keer 2010).

> Educating the patient about the condition is important to encourage a change of lifestyle, where possible, to accommodate the insufficiency of the pelvis. Activities which stress the pelvis should be avoided, such as climbing stairs, one-legged standing, stepping onto a high step, as well as extreme movements of the spine or hip. (Grahame and Keer 2010, p.248)

Gentle pacing of activity with rest is recommended, in keeping with non-HMS women (Tinkle 2010). The other potentially 'better' news for HMS women is that they may fail to develop stretch marks owing to the skin-stretching properties of already lax tissue.

I had major spinal surgery prior to first child. I had pubis symphysis issues and loads of lower back pain and pain into my legs and had to use a wheelchair, so mobility was a real issue. In my second pregnancy my spine was more stable. Pubis symphysis was just as bad, but then arm and shoulder problems worsened. I couldn't get pregnant again – I wouldn't survive physically or mentally. (Anna, aged 37)

Pregnancy – fantastic and no symptoms and had the best time ever. (Sara, aged 34)

LABOUR

There is anecdotal evidence to suggest that the duration of labour is shorter in women with HMS, but there is an increased risk of premature rupture of the membranes or waters breaking. In terms of the delivery, 'it would seem advisable to support the patient's legs and back and prevent excessive unsupported hip abduction' (Grahame and Keer 2010, p.248). Post-delivery there is a greater risk of uterine and genital prolapse in hypermobile women and the potential for developing urinary incontinence. The need to rehabilitate and retrain the pelvic floor muscles is therefore particularly important in the HMS patient (Grahame and Keer 2010; Tinkle 2010).

> The birth itself – I suppose the flexible nature of joints was useful and worked reasonably well, but left the pubic area in a very vulnerable state. Pelvic area was vulnerable and in a mess. (Anna, aged 37)
>
> Birth was very traumatic. I had a terrible time and I had post-partum haemorrhage. Didn't realise this was related to the HMS. Mum who is also hypermobile had the same. (Sara, aged 34)
>
> My pubis symphysis split totally and having an epidural injection didn't work for me and since then I have suffered from chronic back pain because of the epidural. My pelvis was damaged by pregnancy/childbirth and now I walk with sticks or I am confined to a wheelchair. (Becky, aged 27)

MANAGING PARENTHOOD

Since I have not had children, I cannot comment on the experiences of pregnancy or childbirth. I can say that, after spending two days with my gorgeous nine-month-old nephew, I couldn't carry him at all for the rest of the week, but I am assured this becomes easier if you have held them from the beginning, and build up your weight training!

HMS parents had the following comments to make.

Recommendations for HMS pregnancy and parenthood survival

- If you have access to a physio who can advise you on strengthening exercise for areas of vulnerability – get some advice and support.

- Tiredness thing is a huge factor – got to be honest with yourself and ask for help if you need it or you can't survive.

- Was an ardent breast feeder, but I wouldn't advise someone with HMS to do this because it takes so much more out of you nutritionally. You are more likely to have broken nights and physically it is extremely demanding. While it is desirable to breastfeed, you could let yourself off the hook on this matter. You have to look after yourself, or you cannot manage to look after your offspring!

(Anna, aged 37)

I started to get pain at the top of the spine with regard to breast feeding and getting in the right position was difficult. When I was breast feeding my second child, I started getting dislocations again in my left knee probably owing to the hormone prolactin. It is a double-edged sword – I wanted to breast feed but it made my joints worse.

I had problems with carpal tunnel in pregnancy – then as a result of carrying my daughter on my hip (didn't know I had HMS as this point) and trying to carry on and cook dinner I also got tennis elbow from this and ironing, and then I had shoulder and upper back pain, and it has gone up from there. Every day I feel I can't go on and can't cope, but you have to keep going. (Anna, aged 37)

I only became 'HMS' when pregnant and that was the first of my symptoms and pain. When my son was 2 years old, I became housebound. I turned things around by having lots of physio and Pilates was a god-send. It has taken 18 months, and I am still doing it now. I can now do daily activities again and manage children and cleaning, but gardening is too much and it takes me 3–4 days to recover from that. (Jo, aged 27)

MENOPAUSE

As the menopause approaches, the amount of oestrogen and progesterone produced declines rapidly and menstruation ceases. Some women might find that their joints are affected as a result of this change in hormones.

My problems started with periods, which were always extremely painful. In my late teens I started to get dragging stomach pains and tiredness a few days before the start of my period and thought it was PMS related. I went on the pill, which helped a lot, but when I came off in the hope of getting pregnant my symptoms returned. I had a miscarriage but then went on to have our daughter who also has HMS. My pregnancy was fine, but things gradually got much worse afterwards despite being on the pill. I came off the pill and tried other remedies for what was assumed to be PMS but nothing worked and the low stomach pains became constant throughout the month. I eventually had a total hysterectomy aged 44 after my gynaecologist had tried me on every hormone treatment he could think of. This cured my pain but 18 months later my left sacroiliac joint subluxed for the first time. It is unstable and subluxes and I now have muscle wastage. My pelvis is so unstable I am at present having to wear two different types of support belts. If I had known that I had HMS sooner I might have thought twice about having a hysterectomy and I would have understood the need to maintain an ongoing programme of daily exercises. (Jenny, aged 64)

The worst time was my menopause, which was horrible. I was already being a body-worker by then and I was determined to keep off HRT unless I had to – sometimes acupuncture and herbs helped. In desperation I went to my GP and was put on HRT and this solved it. I don't remember sustaining any injuries or problems. However, I put on a lot of weight, I got very depressed about it, I would get irritable and sometimes 'lose it' and then calm down. It felt like it went on forever.

It was possible I did have an injury during that time, but it would have only been about one. It must have been wrist – yes, that's right. After three falls on that wrist, it used to lock when I was working with it. I was convinced I had a wrist bone floating about. All the physios looked at me in disbelief and I did have physiotherapy. The last time my wrist started locking, the physio obtained an X-ray and found a 'floating bone'. After this it never happened again. I felt quite triumphant about this and then this was the end of the episode and it has never bothered me again! (Grace, aged 65)

CONCLUSION

Hormones can have a profound influence on joint and tissue laxity, in particular progesterone prior to menstruation. If you are experiencing a sudden change in your pain levels it might be that hormones are to blame, particularly if you have changed hormone medication, become pregnant, or are going through the menopause! It would be prudent to seek advice if symptoms are suddenly exacerbated.

Conditions such as endometriosis or irregular periods might cause additional difficulties for women with HMS, but advice should be sought in their management from a gynaecologist, as required. The HMSA moderated membership forum might be a good place for further support with respect to pregnancy and birth – see the Resources section at the end of the book.

CHAPTER 9

Psychological Support and HMS

> What can I do? I can't win. People look past it including family and friends who have accused me of getting attention. I just want to be normal and 'not hurt'. Walk a day in my shoes and then you might understand. (Becky, aged 27)

One of the problems about having a hidden disability is other people's reactions, which are often knee-jerk and are based on a lack of empathy or understanding. I spoke to many people with HMS while writing the book and this came up time and time again. Several people mentioned 'walking one day in my shoes' as a way for other people to understand what it is like enduring HMS.

Depression and anxiety are never far away, where HMS is concerned. I have frequently felt like a hypochondriac because of the peculiar way in which injury and pain seem to travel around my body, and how a weekly visit to my physiotherapist will bring up something else. At one point, in 2001, I am sure that the medical profession thought that my pain was psychosomatic. I was being seen by an array of medical professionals including an orthopaedic surgeon, a neurosurgeon, a gynaecologist, a pain management consultant and a gastroenterologist. Interestingly, I was diagnosed with both endometriosis and IBS, and it was the gastroenterologist who showed the most lateral thinking in ensuring I had an MRI of my pelvis (which showed polycystic ovaries) and a spinal MRI (which showed a posterior disc bulge at L4/5). However, the gynaecologist considered my endometriosis 'cured' at that time, the orthopaedic surgeon and neurosurgeon did not consider my back pain as in need of surgery and the orthopaedic surgeon and gynaecologist thought my pain was 'in my mind'. This was incredibly destructive in helping me to get better or to make any improvements to my pain. I met at times with similar attitudes from some family members. This is not at all uncommon and Chapter 7 highlighted the vast range of conditions that are increasingly shown to be related to HMS and how multisystemic it is. It is not therefore surprising that as time went on my mental as well as my physical health began to decline.

> The hardest part is that you know something is wrong and have to fight the medics to be heard. This makes anxiety and depression worse. (Jo, aged 27)

ANXIETY AND HMS

There is increasing evidence to suggest links with anxiety and HMS. People with anxiety disorder were over 16 times more likely than control subjects to have joint laxity. However, there is little evidence to support the fact that panic leads to HMS, so it seems that the HMS condition came first. It is unclear why people with HMS were likely to suffer from anxiety (Martin-Santos *et al.* 1998). However, frequent pain and joint instability might explain why HMS people do exhibit anxiety (Harding 2003; Russek 1999).

A further study found evidence that there is a genetic link between joint hypermobility syndrome and panic (Bulbena *et al.* 2004). State anxiety may be defined as 'feelings of tension and apprehension, associated with arousal of the autonomic nervous system', and trait anxiety refers to 'a general disposition that certain individuals possess to respond to a variety of (relatively unthreatening) situations with high levels of state anxiety' (Hardy, Jones and Gould 1996, p.141). Scores for trait anxiety and to a lesser extent state anxiety were significantly higher for subjects with HMS, suggesting that HMS could be linked to an innate form of excessive response to fear (Bulbena *et al.* 2004). It could be hypothesised that there is something in HMS that leads to anxiety, possibly related to the need to exhibit some control over chaotic tissue laxity. A constant feeling of vulnerability over unstable joints could indeed explain why some HMS patients develop anxiety. However, the following study questions even that point.

A study into the psychological features of HMS in patients who were pain-free at evaluation found that hypermobile subjects were obtaining statistically higher mean scores than the healthy group on all of the nine scales of the SCL-90R Illness Behavior Questionnaire. The SCL-90R scales measure psychological symptoms. The reasons behind these results appear to be linked to the HMS group 'giving more attention to bodily symptoms, perhaps as related to self-perceived weakness and fragility' (Ercolani *et al.* 2008, p.253). There is, it seems, a link between the instability associated with HMS and the range of bodily symptoms, anxiety and general psychological distress. Indeed, it is recommended that physicians should not ignore these symptoms, which might have been dismissed in some HMS patients as hypochondria, and lead to a resentment (from patients) towards the medical profession (Ercolani *et al.* 2008; Grahame 2009a; Harding 2003; Keer 2003).

What is particularly interesting about this study was that the hypermobile group were all asymptomatic and not aware of their diagnosis, and still scored highly on anxiety and other aspects of health psychology behaviour. The fact that the HMS group were not injured suggests that anxiety might be genetically related to HMS. This might imply that anxiety is less relevant in relation to patients (and dancers) who are already injured if, as the literature suggests, the anxiety is already there, perhaps by default (Bulbena *et al.* 2004; Ercolani *et al.* 2008).

Patients at the INPUT Pain Management Centre were given the State Trait Anxiety Inventory (STAI) (Spielberger 1983) but there were no differences between the HMS and non-HMS patients' anxiety scores: 'further work is needed to establish whether the anxiety is a primary feature of HMS, or secondary feature of having a long-term, painful unexplained condition' (Harding 2003, p.150).

In many ways it is no wonder that people with HMS suffer from anxiety. It is constantly difficult being in a body that feels chaotic and out of control. Frequently, I don't know where I am, proprioceptively. A Pilates instructor describes this perfectly: 'this sense of not knowing where you are in space is basically eroding a sense of identity and not knowing who and where you are literally, which makes the condition so debilitating' (Mary, personal communication, 21 May 2010). Although it may be true that HMS shares some of the genetic bases of anxiety, the poor proprioception and physical instability caused by tissue laxity must contribute. Furthermore, some aspects of HMS seem to mimic post-traumatic stress disorder (PTSD), and my investigations for this book led me to reflect on some of the comments of Babette Rothschild in her book *The Body Remembers*. Further research would be necessary in relation to HMS, but these feelings (personally) seem incredibly familiar.

> People with PTSD live with a chronic state of Autonomic Nervous System – ANS activation – hyper-arousal – in their bodies, leading to physical symptoms that are the basis of anxiety, panic, weakness, exhaustion, muscle stiffness, concentration problems and sleep disturbance... It is a vicious cycle... Symptoms can become chronic or can be triggered acutely. Breaking this cycle is an important step in the treatment of PTSD. (Rothschild 2000, p.47)

However, at another level, anxiety for HMS patients will also be about concerns about family and friends, fear of pain and worsening symptoms and even about managing to work and 'have a life'.

PAIN AND DEPRESSION

> You start to believe it, that the pain is in your head, then depression kicks in. When you see someone (a doctor) who understands it, it is like the light comes on and you are not alone. (Becky, aged 27)

There is a proverb, 'a life lived in fear is a life half-lived', and yet many hypermobile patients do live their lives in fear – of pain increasing and being able to do less, and the detrimental effect that this has on themselves, their family and friends:

> HMS is a disorder that robs patients of control over their lives. All chronic illness and chronic pain cause feelings of loss of control. The problem is exacerbated with HMS because there is not always a clear link between an activity and the onset of pain. (Gurley-Green 2001, p.488)

Being in pain is fatiguing, lonely and depressing. Mood can have an impact upon pain and explains the potential value of CBT in order to help. The techniques of pacing, goal-setting and relaxation are also critical in coping with pain (see Chapter 6). Fear, anxiety and depression are made worse when one doesn't know how long something is going to last, or when the last attempt at physical exercise, or even doing something like cleaning or cooking, makes things much worse. It can be very self-defeating. I think it is really important to focus on any achievements, however tiny. Conversely, I know how I feel at the end of a day at work when my back has been 'killing me' and I am too exhausted to process a conversation and all I want is quiet, my bed and a painkiller. If this happens I know how quickly I become anxious that tomorrow will be as bad again, or that I will be completely unproductive. I believe in taking one day at a time. Everyone will have their own way of coping, and I wouldn't want to be prescriptive. However, knowing who you can obtain support from is very important, and appropriately, when!

FAMILY AND FRIENDS

A couple of years ago I went to Legoland with a friend of mine and her mother. By the time we had walked from the car park to the entrance I was knackered and done for the day. I ended up trailing round after them, getting further and further behind and missing half the park as I just didn't have the energy to drag myself any further. (Jo Anne, aged 41)

People look at you like you are lazy and cannot be bothered. I was accused of being a lazy teenager by an old man who saw me in an electric mobility scooter. (Becky, aged 27)

One of the huge negatives in a deceptively hidden disability is that patients look well, which makes it difficult to convince others that there is a problem. This is even worse with HMS because our sometimes 'amazing' mobility can seriously detract from the pain and difficulties that many of us endure daily. Many HMSA members that I talked to say that, even when their mobility declines to an extent, the pain and symptoms actively remain (Gurley-Green 2001). The lack of sympathy and understanding by some family members and friends is something that as a group HMSA patients are unfortunately used to. Thoughtless comments are frequently deeply upsetting and show an ignorance of the plight of the difficulties and pain that HMSA patients regularly endure. It can be hard to shake off such comments and it is upsetting and frustrating. After all, if our closest family members do not believe us, what hope do we have with friends, employers and the medical profession?

CONVINCING THE MEDICAL PROFESSION

Everyone has to fight to get a diagnosis, and to cope with not being diagnosed by the medical profession. Then depression goes with all of that. It is an invisible illness. The hardest part is that you know something is wrong and have to fight the medics to be heard. This makes anxiety and depression worse. (Jo, aged 27)

Most HMSA members have their own story in terms of their battles with the medical profession in accepting their HMS seriously. Far too many of us will have been told our pain is psychosomatic and we often have to see many different consultants before we are finally given a diagnosis. It takes a particularly astute medical consultant to make a diagnosis, and HMS does involve some detective work if one does not know or understand what to look for. It is not surprising that many of us become frustrated with the medical profession until the time of diagnosis. However, some of us have been fortunate to have been seen at NHS hospitals where the Rheumatology Department has an expertise in HMS such as University College Hospital in London (UCH) with Professor Rodney Grahame. When you finally speak to and see a consultant who understands HMS, it is really wonderful and helps to finally understand all the previous problems we have endured and why it is so likely to be linked to having HMS.

Professors Rodney Grahame, Howard Bird and William Ferrell and Dr Alan Hakim have done enormous amounts in order to educate the medical profession and to encourage them to 'think outside the box' with HMS, which is why links are being made with other conditions and HMS – for example, gut motility problems. One of the best outcomes of writing this book would be to educate other medical professionals about the condition so that future generations will not have to wait so long to get the help they so crucially deserve. I do hope that all rheumatology and physiotherapy departments will have access to this book. As information about HMS circulates (the Internet is an excellent place to start), people at all levels will become better informed and then my hope would be for funding to be found in order to research improved treatment outcomes and perhaps even genetic modifications into our faulty collagens one day in the future. I also hope that one resultant outcome of normal collagens would be higher energy levels so I could manage more of a social life!

SOCIAL LIFE

I cannot go out drinking. I am 21 years of age. I have only been clubbing three times this year – the pain is just unbearable. It is really hard explaining this to friends. (Bobbie, aged 21)

There are occasions when I like to have things planned out in my diary so I can see what I have coming up and to avoid doing too much, but there are other occasions when springing something 'unplanned' on me is much better. When I am in fatigue mode, looking at my diary and seeing several evenings out can sometimes just seem too much on top of the working day, even when it is friends that I really want to see. I have cancelled or postponed so many social events that I wonder how I have any friends or social life left at all, yet this really isn't social avoidance as much as pacing and surviving a chronic condition which doesn't take into account that occasionally I need to have fun and enjoy myself. To any of my friends and family who are reading this, I can only apologise and wish things were a bit different, but thank you for being there just the same and coping with the inevitable postponed evenings out. I prefer going out on good form as opposed to completely collapsed or in pain. I appreciate your continued efforts to invite me out and, as I say, sometimes the unplanned or last-minute events are often the best because I am caught unawares and, if I am 'good to go', I will!

One of the most difficult social events are ones where I am required to stand a lot as in a drinks party, or long theatre sessions when I cannot fidget. I remember going to see a play and I had to leave halfway through because the seats were too uncomfortable. I have similarly left cinemas and other shows because I was in too much pain. At drinks parties, even the alcohol doesn't help (much); it is just that it requires a lot more effort to stand still because it is so much harder to control our range of movement when not moving through the joint. I find art galleries difficult because it is too 'stop-start' and I fatigue very quickly. I manage now by just doing very short visits to galleries and at drinks parties I move about, sitting down when necessary. However, it feels embarrassing needing to sit down when there are frequently older people than myself who manage perfectly well. I have also been given a hard time on public transport when I have occasionally asked for a seat.

Shopping used to be a great challenge before the advent of online shopping. I now get a food shopping delivery to my home at least every one or two months of all the heavier items so I don't have to carry them. This is also a pacing strategy I was seriously asked to consider as part of my pain management and to help my back pain. I have never been a very serious shopper, and in terms of clothes shopping give up quickly if I can't find what I am looking for, but I have been assured by non-HMS people there is nothing abnormal about that anyway.

I believe that the pacing of activities was one of the most useful practical learning outcomes I gained from attending the pain management course, and this really is crucial with HMS. It is not good for people with HMS to sit in prolonged positions, and many HMS patients don't cope with overuse or repetitive movements. It is important to occasionally fidget or change positions and this might be particularly crucial in having intimate relationships.

INTIMATE RELATIONSHIPS

Having had a thorough look at a particular thread on the HMSA online (closed membership) forum, it seemed that my own experiences in the bedroom were little short of normal (for a hypermobile person) – minus the dislocations, which I am fortunate enough not to sustain. It seems to be 'standard' to feel wiped out after sexual intercourse, however brief the encounter, and to have back and hip pain, which is commonly reported. Some members had difficulties with skin tearing, which is another unfortunate and painful result of excessive tissue laxity. Ways forward for managing tearing and vaginal dryness included ensuring the use of adequate lubrication and condoms that were more sensitive and less likely to cause irritation or allergy. Some members suggested the use of cushions for comfort and changing positions regularly to avoid discomfort and overuse and to minimise the pain, especially that caused by deep penetration. Many members advocated the essentials of having a good sense of humour and a very sensitive and loving partner. A number of other members added to the thread by saying 'What sex life?', while other posts confirmed that sex caused too much pain or fatigue to contemplate. For others their hypermobility was occasionally an advantage in the bedroom, but many advocated that sexual activity often resulted in increased pain and fatigue and that they didn't have it too often for that reason. Some members pointed out the perils of oral sex where dislocating their jaws became an issue, while other members thought that the Rampant Rabbit should be available on NHS prescription! The need for good communication was highlighted as paramount in terms of intimate relationships, and an understanding and loving partner.

The longevity of a relationship is likely to be tested to the limit when one partner has a chronic and painful condition. It is hard living with someone day in and day out who is sometimes unable to work, who is regularly in pain and unable to do much, and is sometimes so fatigued they cannot remember their own postcode! While some relationships inevitably survive, many do not. In the end I left my last partner as I felt it was unfair to continue to inflict my depression on them. The relationship had probably died long before then, but although my physical situation didn't decline any more rapidly, my mental health declined detrimentally, including an aborted attempt at taking my own life. If a bottom point was reached, or if I had sunk to my lowest ebb, it was probably between 2005 and 2006. I had gained a lot of weight, I was barely working, and I did nothing. I watched TV. I did nothing else. I saw hardly anyone and I wanted to sleep a lot. I was no longer in love with my partner, but I had no love for myself at all. I saw no point in continuing to live and at one point I literally hoped that I would die and that the lights would all go out.

SELF-HARM IN HMS AND OTHER CHRONIC CONDITIONS

Although there is no documented research that I could find linking HMS and self-harm, there were postings on the topic on the HMSA online forum, and anecdotally the medical liaison officer at the HMSA told me that she had heard many stories from adolescents and even children who felt suicidal because of their condition. This is a grave state of affairs and the emotional impact of a condition that frequently leaves the sufferer so unstable because of their chaotic tissue laxity must be further investigated. Spanish research into anxiety and panic is very telling (Martin-Santos *et al.* 1998). When I first emailed the medical liaison officer at the HMSA and she told me about how common self-harm was (anecdotally), I felt extremely sad through my own long history of self-harm which I eventually chose to publicly document through poetry (*The Skin Collection*, Knight 2009b). My self-harm involved skin picking and I have some serious scars which can now only reflect my despair. I started to harm myself from the very young age of 5 and I think that the reason I felt so sad when I heard about other HMSA patients harming was because it was just another piece of the jigsaw that slotted into place in terms of my own personal journey with HMS since diagnosis. People self-harm to escape very difficult feelings, such as anxiety and depression, but I frequently remember having this sensation of feeling at odds with my body, feeling disconnected with it, that it felt 'unreal' not knowing where I was and feeling out of control, which I think might just link to having a very poor sense of proprioception. I would have self-harmed to 'get back into' and connect with my body. Seeing blood and mess and then sensing pain helped me to regain control. I can only join the dots now. I self-harmed for 27 years before finally obtaining the right psychological support for me. Having tried cognitive behavioural therapy as a teenager, which didn't work for me, and then psychotherapy, which also didn't work for me personally, I was referred for cognitive analytical therapy (CAT), which really helped me. Although I do have occasional blips, I manage far more successfully now. The Association for Cognitive Analytical Therapy (ACAT) defines CAT:

> Cognitive Analytic Therapy involves a therapist and a client working together to look at what has hindered changes in the past, in order to understand better how to move forward in the present.

Questions like 'Why do I always end up feeling like this?' become more answerable. (ACAT 2011)

One of the first things I did with Dr H (my CAT therapist) was to identify the different moods that I could get into that caused me to feel uncomfortable and then ultimately self-harm. When I became quite good at this, we looked at how I could get into different states with people – perhaps feeling controlled, or angry, and then I would turn to self-harm as a way of dealing with this feeling rather than discussing it directly with the other person.

In addition to that, it was also noted that I could go into a completely numb and detached state which was when the self-harm often took place. One of the most important aspects of the therapy was to involve me getting back in touch with my real physical body and all its sensations: the good and the bad. This was particularly hard for me given that I suffer from two chronic and frequently very painful conditions called HMS and endometriosis. (Isobel Knight)

If the past few paragraphs have struck a chord with you, I would urge you to get the appropriate psychological support that you deserve. Please visit your GP or discuss with a member of your medical team. If you are ever feeling very distressed please do not wait to harm yourself before getting urgent support. The Samaritans are invaluable if you are not able to talk to a friend, family member or GP first. My hope through writing my own story of self-harm is not only that this topic will be brought out in the open but also that the medical profession will seek, within the realms of available resources, to better support those of us who have chronic conditions. There is a general lack of emotional and psychological support in managing HMS and other chronic conditions, other than what is offered within the realms of pain management, but it is just not enough.

SUPPORT IN PSYCHOLOGICAL MANAGEMENT

So far this chapter has discussed some of the known psychological links with HMS and anxiety as well as coping with the difficulties of a chronic condition in terms of friends and family, the medical profession, social

149

support and within intimate relationships. Mention has been made in this chapter (and Chapter 6) of depression but so far less has been mentioned in terms of other ways of obtaining support. Psychological support via CBT, CAT and psychotherapy has been mentioned, and there are online forums such as the HMSA Forum, which is carefully moderated. There are also HMSA groups that meet regionally and more can be found in the Resources section. Talking has a crucial place in communicating difficult feelings, and knowing who to turn to in terms of family or friends is important, but there are times when seeking the support of a professional is essential. There is also drug therapy which for many can be invaluable in improving their psychological health. There is an essential place for antidepressants, some of which have a dual role in helping with depression and chronic pain, for example Amitriptyline (there is further information on drugs in Chapter 6). Relaxation (see Chapter 6) might also help with resultant anxiety and meditation. Some complementary therapies have been known to help with anxiety and depression, although further evidence-based research is required in order to verify this. Therapies that might be worth considering for this purpose include Reiki, Bowen therapy, Shiatsu and massage. This chapter concludes by looking at the psychology and economics of managing a chronic condition and managing to work with HMS and welfare benefit assistance.

MANAGING AT WORK

The Job Centre have said I am not a viable option for an employer. I am now studying psychology and training to be a teacher and might go into research work in the future. (Becky, aged 27)

My own feelings concerning my career are that I am about ten years behind where I wanted to be in real time through my HMS and endometriosis. Since 2001, I have been unable to manage a conventionally full-time 9am to 5pm Monday to Friday job. In the past year I have probably been working a six-day week, but the intensity of it varies. I have come to the conclusion that having a variety of jobs (I do three) seems to suit me better, physically and psychologically, than doing a conventional working week. Even though many people think that I have achieved highly both academically and professionally, I cannot see this because I still feel disappointed in my overall career and I have experienced significant financial loss through lack of work, or being unable to manage to work at a full-time conventional post. Even though financial status should not reflect professional status, in our society it unfortunately seems to, and therefore according to that law, I have generally 'failed'. On another level I have perhaps been highly successful and my determination has seen me through on many occasions. I have just had to find a different way to manage to work and to support myself. I still feel angry that this is the case and I am frustrated that I have not been able to do certain things and find too many obstacles in where I presently want to go owing to lack of available funding. I am thinking here of research into HMS. Even after completing this book I hope that I can continue with some of my academic endeavours and future writing and research into HMS.

In 2001 I had a long period of absences from work and stopped working in full-time posts from that point onward. I just remember waking every day and being far too exhausted and in too much pain to work. When I got to work I was little short of useless because I was too fatigued to concentrate and in too much pain to manage anything. The post I managed to obtain by the end of 2001 was a part-time post as a volunteer manager, and gave me a good salary rise so that I was almost on (part time) what I had formerly been on full time as an administrator. It was a good result and at the time I was living with my partner, and so had their financial help. I could pace my week so long as I worked on Mondays – and so I could afford some flexibility if I had a very bad day, or needed to change working days. For me this worked very well. There is no doubt that a sympathetic boss is vital in order to successfully manage to work.

In 2002 I decided to train as a Bowen therapist. The Bowen technique had generally been instrumentally helpful with my back pain and in helping with my own wellbeing. I was so impressed with this subtle and seemingly 'simple' technique that I decided to train as a therapist. All I can say is more fool me, because Bowen is actually very difficult to learn and even harder to perform it well considering its deceptively simple and hands-off approach. I experienced great difficulties in learning it which I would now link to the possibilities of being dyspraxic and problems with memory and sequential learning (see Chapter 4). I qualified in 2003 and I believe because of my struggles to learn to do Bowen well I have actually, and to my complete surprise, probably become a very good therapist because I had to work harder to learn it. Bowen is wonderful in terms of my HMS because the frequent breaks in the treatment mean I can rest and there is no danger of overuse as there is with massage. It is gentle on the therapist as well as the patient. Bowen still forms an important part of my week; I practise both from home and at Trinity Laban at the Laban Health Clinic (a leading conservatoire for music and dance based in South London), and so one of my dreams of working with dancers has been realised.

In 2003 my (then) partner and I left London to live in Cambridge. I left the job as a volunteer manager, and successfully obtained a very similar post in Cambridge, but didn't take it on owing to severe depression at the time. This was a big mistake, because while I was setting up practice as a Bowen therapist, I had no other form of income, and at this point started to do less and less. I then got some part-time work in telesales and, as my depression gradually deepened, my confidence lessened and I felt I was only just about 'good enough' to do telesales work, although I was still doing some Bowen. One of my clinics did very well, but then the clinic closed and the other practices I worked at never really took off in the same way. Subsequently my mood deteriorated, I became less and less active (I had been doing Pilates and swimming regularly from 2001 to 2003) and then I virtually ground to a halt on all fronts until I made the huge decision to leave my partner and return to London. This decision probably saved my life.

In early 2006 I returned to London. I started to do some Bowen work in a new clinic and found some supporting telesales work. I did the telesales work for a month and then wanted to leave as I hated it so much, and then I wasn't paid for all my work. This was almost the final straw for me. I had no money; I was in debt and was now supporting myself. I had a long court battle with the telesales employer, and was finally reimbursed at the end of 2007. I was very fortunate in that my grandmother gave me some money which allowed me to stay on in London. I had another spell at this point on benefits as I was psychologically very unstable at this point, and my HMS and endometriosis were also very severe. Two things which helped were attending the residential pain management course in September 2006 and then having CAT therapy to help with the depression and self-harm. A part-time post as a volunteer manager came up with a lovely charity enabling adults with disabilities to visit art galleries and museums. It was a 14 hour per week post and with the Bowen work was just enough for me to cope with. In many ways that job helped me successfully back on my feet and rebuilt my shattered confidence. By 2007 I was doing 21 hours per week for the charity and had a busy Bowen clinic one day per week. My financial situation and security improved my self-confidence and my self-esteem improved; I felt more in control of my life in all sorts of ways. I had also started dancing again and this in turn was improving my fitness and mood (see Chapters 6 and 10).

In 2008 I started my MSc in Dance Science, and was managing that around 16 hours at the charity job and some Bowen work (I had cut this down to help with the course). I was literally working seven days per week either studying or actively working. It was a massive but exhausting turn-around.

Having completed my MSc I continued to work at the charity 16 hours per week until the charity was sadly shut down in March 2010. I worked 14 hours per week at Trinity Laban as the clinic admin manager and was doing two days per week of Bowen and academic research. Once I was made redundant from the charity job, I retrenched that time to write this book. They say that life is never dull, and the last two years certainly haven't been. I never thought I would achieve this, given my situation particularly between 2000 and 2006. As my confidence and ability grows and the way I can often cope with my HMS improves, I am probably raising the bar even higher. I believe that my future might lie in health journalism and writing alongside Bowen work and academic research and/or some form of management. I do use life coaching skills such as self-talk and mental imaging to imagine where I want to be and find this helpful. I will still not commit to a conventional post because of my medical conditions and because I hate letting people down. I might be a lot stronger and fitter in a musculoskeletal capacity than I have ever been before, but no amount of physiotherapy or Bowen is sadly going to help with the fatigue, and for that reason alone I will not return to full-time work. I must not feel a failure because I cannot manage this. I am very lucky to manage what I am doing now; there are so many HMS patients who are in a much worse state than I am now in and for them work can only remain a dream. I have to say that, for those who can manage something, voluntary work is a wonderful way in which to start. I have supported many volunteers with depression who have found that doing voluntary work was a positive and safe way in which to consider returning to doing any kind of work. Of course I am realistic that not everyone can comprehend managing work, and having had two episodes on benefits, I am very aware of the essential need for welfare benefits.

OBTAINING SUPPORT – WELFARE BENEFITS

The very worst thing is that I cannot get any kind of disability benefit (although I do manage to qualify for disability tax credits but only because I was on long-term incapacity before I got my present part-time job) because nothing I have gets me an automatic tick in a box. They don't seem to understand that the cumulative effect of all three 'minor' problems adds up to a poor quality of life. (Jo Anne, aged 41)

In the UK, the government's budget (June 2010) has shown cuts in the welfare benefits system that could affect those who need them most. It is perhaps good to have benefits removed from those who have no need for them or play the system, but few people want to be on incapacity benefit unless they need to have it and it is extremely hard that they have to spend time and energy convincing the powers that be that they are in serious need of the benefit in order to survive. It is hard enough managing a chronic condition without having to fight for continued economic survival. The changes that the UK government are making are still unfolding, but it seems that as always it will be difficult for those in particular need, which is so grossly unjust.

Seeing an occupational therapist at your workplace or within an NHS setting might be helpful in a paced and gradual return to work. Your physiotherapist can give advice on aspects such as overuse syndrome at work and taking care to avoid repetitive movements. Advice can also be obtained on the use of splints such as wrist splints, if required to help at work. Organisations such as Access to Work can be helpful and might, for example, contribute towards taxi fares for work, an improved desk station and other work-related practical assistance, such as adapting equipment.

CONCLUSION

This chapter has looked at the psychological dimension of managing HMS. It has covered:

- anxiety and HMS
- pain and depression
- family and friends
- convincing the medical profession
- social life
- intimate relationships
- self-harm in HMS and other chronic conditions
- support in psychological management
- managing at work
- obtaining support – welfare benefits.

It will always be difficult for those of us who live with unseen medical conditions, especially HMS where the individual looks apparently healthy and well. It is hard to continue deflecting insensitive comments and to have to 'convince' someone that you are in pain. For that reason people with HMS need great personal inner strength and a sense of humour helps. It is psychologically draining to continue to fight with a condition where control and stability are an enigma and a whole myriad of other related symptoms form part of daily life. 'Walk one day in my shoes and then you'll understand…'

CHAPTER 10

Dancers and HMS

If you are a non-dancer, please do not skip this chapter because much of the information applied to dancers can equally be applied to non-dancers!

> On being hypermobile: 'It is like my best friend and my worst enemy – but I wouldn't wish it on anyone and wouldn't give it away!' (Zinzi Minot, contemporary dance student, Trinity Laban)

Hypermobility is highly prevalent within the dance sector; up to 70 per cent particularly within the ballet and contemporary dance community are hypermobile, compared to 10–30 per cent within the non-dance population. One of the key components of dance is flexibility and the ability to produce aesthetically pleasing postures (Figure 10.1), often at the end range of normal joint movement. Joint hypermobility has been documented as advantageous during the selection process for a career in dance, while some dancers acquire hypermobility by virtue of their training in order to produce the beautiful extensions that many choreographers require (Desfor 2003; Liederbach 2000; McCormack *et al.* 2004; Ruemper 2008).

It seems that the artistic and aesthetic components of hypermobility might be considered as its main value in dance and 'performance arts', since there is also a prevalence in musicians, gymnastics and acrobatics (Bird 2007b; Desfor 2003). The ability to be able to 'stretch' the body into unusual and interesting shapes is of interest to choreographers in dancers and for musicians it might be advantageous to have hypermobility of the hands in order to more easily manage some composers' works. For example, it is likely that Sergei Rachmaninoff and Niccolò Paganini were hypermobile because of the extensive ranges in their music. The high prevalence of hypermobility in the performing arts sector suggests that people with hypermobility are drawn to this area of work and artistry because they are naturally good at it. If dancers have generalised hypermobility, which is hypermobility that is asymptomatic and not causing pain, they are much more likely to manage a successful dance career. In an informal discussion about hypermobile dancers, a Trinity Laban classical ballet teacher with over 30 years of experience commented: 'The advantages of hypermobility are extensions and lines and line of leg and arabesque. That would be the main thing – that the line is more pleasing, but then there appear to be more disadvantages than advantages' (Teresa Kelsey, personal communication, 13 May 2010).

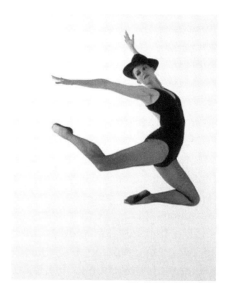

Figure 10.1: Mari Frogner,
contemporary dancer
Photo by Alicia Clarke

Some dancers acquire some of their hypermobility through training. 'Acquired hypermobility' when measuring elite gymnasts (who are warmed up) shows an appreciable loss within 15–20 minutes at the end of training when the body is cool again (Bird, Walker and Newton 1988). Dancers with GJH could have a very successful career with no increased risk of injury compared to the non-hypermobile dancer. However, dancers with HMS are less likely to get to the top because of pain and regular injuries and there is a correlation between injury and HMS within dancers in the contemporary dance population (Desfor 2003; Liederbach 2000; Ruemper 2008).

> A key finding…was a decrease in prevalence of JHS in ascending from junior school, through the senior school to Company, and within the Company from Corps de Ballet to principal dancer. We suggested that JHS may be associated with a greater risk of injury and/or prolonged periods of recovery post-injury, which may have an adverse effect on career development. (Briggs *et al.* 2009, p.1469)

Once a dancer with HMS becomes injured, the chances of further injury are very likely, but it is unclear whether injuries in HMS dancers take longer to heal, or whether there is greater tissue damage before injury, or both. It seems likely that the collagen deficiency may mean that the tissues are already weaker, leaving HMS dancers more open to injury. Early identification and intervention is important in HMS dancers in order to prevent injury (Briggs *et al.* 2009).

In my case it was probably just as well I didn't have my heart set on becoming a professional dancer because, unless I had received much earlier diagnosis and intervention, I would have been unlikely to succeed because of my HMS (aside from a lack of natural talent!). I would certainly not want to put off any dancers reading this chapter, but research clearly shows that HMS ballet dancers seem less likely to make it to the very top of their career, although they may still succeed at having fulfilled careers in dance performance (Briggs *et al.* 2009). In the contemporary dance sector this might be different, and more research would need to be conducted to look at HMS contemporary dancers who are still successfully performing. There is a clear correlation between HMS and injury in contemporary dance (Ruemper 2008), but my hope is that despite their HMS there are still many dancers managing to dance. It would be interesting to find out whether they are managing to dance because they just happened to have avoided injury, or because they are following good intervention plans, or both. The incidents of HMS in other styles of dance are not well documented since flexibility is not an essential aesthetical component in some dance styles such as hip hop, tap dance and flamenco. This chapter mainly concentrates on those who are engaged in either classical ballet or contemporary dance.

I am now dancing again despite all the odds, the pain and increased injury risk. Why? Because I love dancing and it is a chance to use my range of movement and flexibility to its full advantage, coupled with the fact it is the only form of exercise I truly enjoy. Ballet classes coupled with regular Pilates and physiotherapy are keeping me well conditioned. The better physically conditioned I am, the less pain I am in and the stronger my muscles remain, supporting my large range of movement. I would never advocate someone stopping something they truly enjoy, but I would want them to be realistic about the difficulties they are more likely to encounter because of their joint laxity and related symptoms. However, the power of the mind is a wonderful thing and that combined with bloody-mindedness and a characteristic stubborn streak are what keep me going in all sorts of ways and keep me at the barre.

CHARACTERISTICS OF HYPERMOBILE DANCERS

Anecdotal evidence suggests that it might be possible to recognise hypermobile dancers by virtue of their behaviour. Figure 10.2 depicts a dancer with a hypermobile spine, hanging in forward flexion, before going into prolonged stretches (Batson 1992, p.42). A ballet teacher commented on hypermobile dancers: 'Their sense of spatial awareness appears under-developed, they have a tendency to lack proprioception, they have difficulty in sensing their dynamic alignment and their concentration can be inconsistent and their focus dispersed' (Teresa Kelsey, personal communication, 9 June 2009). Studying an adolescent dance population, I tried to see whether there were significant differences in the anxiety and perfectionist scores between injured and non-injured HMS dancers and, while there were no significant differences between these two groups, there were differences between HMS dancers and non-HMS dancers in terms of perfectionism scores, with HMS dancers scoring significantly higher, suggesting that they perhaps have to work twice as hard by virtue of their HMS, although these are only preliminary findings (Knight 2009a).

Further research is looking at the learning and behavioural characteristics of HMS dancers since it has been noticed anecdotally that

HMS dancers seem to process things differently in a learning capacity, and that they do not always seem to be in time with the music. As Teresa Kelsey comments, 'Hypermobile dancers can be either slightly behind or ahead of the music. I don't know whether this is because of the thinking process in what they are trying to achieve physically, but they do not always keep to the tempo of the music' (personal communication, 13 May 2010). Research has shown links with HMS and DCD (see Chapter 4) so it might be that HMS dancers do have different learning needs, but the evidence is presently too insubstantial. Further research is required to make connections with HMS and other learning difficulties, for example dyslexia and attention deficit disorder. Despite the sophisticated level of motor control required in dance, it would be most interesting to observe whether dancers with hypermobility have any perceived difficulty in motor coordination and in 'learning' dance. Perhaps it is the case that learning dance has helped hypermobile dancers overcome coordination difficulties.

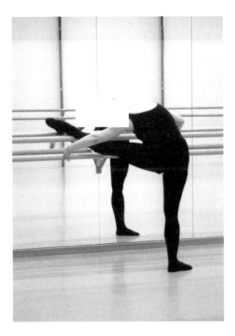

Figure 10.2: HMS dancer 'hanging into forward flexion' and 'into her joints' at the barre

WHAT IS GOOD ABOUT BEING A HYPERMOBILE DANCER?

Hypermobile dancers might be perceived to behave differently – for example going into prolonged stretches (Batson 1992), perhaps just because they can – so why is hypermobility an advantageous aspect to the dancer?

What is good about being hypermobile is the range of movement you have – not just in legs, but in the back. I have more reach and can make myself look bigger – even though I am quite short. I have more space to use. It gives the ability to do things with my body that I can achieve regardless of being a dancer and my training, which is what is nice. It belongs to me. Nobody can have it. If they don't, if they do, then… Got it! Great! (Zinzi Minot, contemporary dance student, Trinity Laban)

I was a very gifted performer because I was so sensitive and supple and I could make all these beautiful shapes – my back is extremely supple. (Mary, Pilates instructor and former dancer)

The remainder of the chapter focuses on the disadvantages and difficulties experienced by hypermobile dancers, solutions and ways forward.

DIFFICULTIES FOR HYPERMOBILE DANCERS

The following difficulties would be similar and likely for all dancers with generalised hypermobility, which is hypermobility that is asymptomatic, and therefore advantageous to dance, as well as for those with HMS, and this corresponds with the list set out in Chapter 2. However, these listed difficulties are resultant difficulties from HMS, so in this chapter we start to look at managing the resultant difficulties (described in detail in Chapter 2) in relation to dancers. The main difficulties are:

- pain (widespread and localised)
- fatigue
- joint pain

- regular soft-tissue trauma

- dislocations and subluxations

- slow healing

- overuse injuries.

One of the biggest problems for dancers and other patients with HMS is a lack of strength to match their large range of movement and flexibility. Addressing this is going to be critical to managing other related difficulties.

Figure 10.3 shows how improving strength fits in as another part of the strategy which would be to improve proprioceptive control. Once dancers and other people with HMS start to have these attributes coupled with such pain management strategies as pacing employed in Chapter 6, it is just possible that pain might improve and that injury rates decline because of improved strength and proprioception. However, dancers and other individuals will need a good deal of support from a dance/HMS physiotherapist specialist and Pilates instructor coupled with being overseen by a physician or consultant rheumatologist, where appropriate.

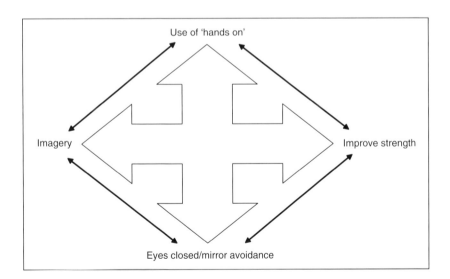

Figure 10.3: Strategies for improving proprioception

If I could have done my career over again I would say I would have to have had daily input from Pilates teachers which I didn't. I needed much more strength because I was over-supple. I did have weekly physio, which helped me a lot and kept me on the road. Hypermobile dancers can go into a career but they have to have a tremendous amount of help of body-workers and Pilates to balance them out and strength in the right place. Pilates is one of the few complementary and holistic approaches that looks at the musculoskeletal side of things, the energetic picture and the emotional side of things. It just really balances people out very well without being too 'woolly' to work on the musculoskeletal imbalances. It can work on the local as well as the global imbalances and you can work on the hypermobile joints and you can mobilise joints that have become short-locked because of other parts of the fascia being too long-locked. And it is a very good way of keeping your individual needs in the picture. Yoga is very good but yoga is more global and doesn't work on specific joints, and yoga is usually conducted in a group whereas Pilates is one to one. (Mary, Pilates instructor)

MY EXPERIENCES OF RETURNING TO CLASSICAL BALLET AND INJURY

My return to classical ballet classes was the result of starting to understand the message that 'pain doesn't always equal damage' which I first heard while on the pain management course that I attended in 2006. So how did I return to ballet classes? Initially I did pace myself. It was frustrating because my brain remembered the steps, and there was definitely plenty of muscular memory, but my body was significantly deconditioned at the beginning and it was very hard for me in making the mental leap that I had to cope with my legs being very low, and my control was simply extremely poor. I felt trapped in the wrong body. I returned to classes with Teresa Kelsey in central London, doing both her (then) pre-elementary and elementary classes. However, from my diary entries it appears that I only stuck to doing ballet classes from September 2006, until approximately April 2007, and then I stopped again.

Towards the end of 2007 I started dancing again in the privacy of my own home and this possibly kept me conditioned just sufficiently enough and then I decided to start ballet classes again from January 2008, once or twice a week. At this point I probably went completely mad and threw all caution to the wind. My diary suggests that I went from doing little bits of ballet at home to five classes per week with no pacing or particular intelligence. The mere concept of 'periodisation' – the planning of physical activity, pacing and training – was completely absent. I was dancing again almost from zero to doing several classes per week. I thought my body was ready for it and that it could take it, but fairly quickly old problems arose – low back pain, calf overuse, systemic pain – all the things that in fact unbeknown to me were totally HMS related, in a deconditioned body, and then I injured myself significantly. I clearly remember going to the ballet class and in my logical brain knowing I shouldn't be there, but here was a case of passion outweighing logic. I needed to be at that class, because if I wasn't I wouldn't continue to gain fitness, I might just deteriorate, and so despite immense fatigue and extremely sore calves, I attended this class with a different teacher from normal. I went for it despite the pain and during *assemblés* (jumps where two feet meet in the air) I heard my calf physically tear and I knew it was all going to be over for some time.

The poem I wrote to explain my calf tear probably does so more aptly than I can now.

Breaking Point

I should have known it was going to happen
The day before I felt the warning signals;
A siren beeping in my leg
Just a minute!

In one space I am dancing fantastically,
My body is responding beautifully to all the instructions
Fluent, free-flowing and seamless sequences
My whole form extended in curvaceous lines.
Then.

It just snapped. I heard the tear.

The end grounded me, and I swept my body from the floor.

Pain seared in my calf, and I just wanted to howl.

All I could see was the wall and weeks of no ballet.

It is the end of the world, and is so unfair.

People crowd around who care, but they are really thinking, 'thank God it wasn't me'

My life changed in one second.

The point that broke my leg.

(© Isobel Knight 2009b)

Quite soon after the injury, I started a blog which was a way of diarising my recovery from the injury. What I never, ever anticipated at the time was that I would still be rehabilitating my body over two years later. (See Knight 2008–2010; the blog is still continuing.)

My initial blog entries are shown in the box.

Sunday, 10 February 2008: visit to A&E

I had already applied ice to my calf and waited to be seen with more ice and some painkillers. I couldn't take any weight on my leg and although have strained the very same muscle groups many times over, I had never done so to this extent and was concerned about how badly I had done it since I heard the tear.

I was given crutches and told to keep my weight off the leg and was discharged with further painkillers and told to return to A&E should my calf suddenly swell up or become anymore painful (difficult to imagine) in case I had a DVT. It was now no longer considered necessary or beneficial to bandage or Tubigrip the calf in case of blood clots, although the human in me very much wanted to do just that.

Some kind friends picked me up from A&E and drove me home and I sat and ate pizza (the only thing I could easily bung in the oven) and pondered the news I wouldn't be dancing for at least 4–6 weeks.

Before I went to bed I gave myself a Bowen treatment and did the knee procedure on myself, the most logical one to attempt given all the moves on the calf muscles. I elevated my leg on a pillow and tried to sleep, negotiating the cat. It was not a happy night.

Monday, 11 February 2008

I took a taxi to hospital today so I could see the 'acute' physiotherapy.

The main thing that took place at that session was the physio ensuring that I walked normally as soon as possible and not walk on my toes which she said would store up trouble later on. It was suggested I could wear high-heels as this would take pressure off my calf. Reader, I can just see that happening. I don't own anything with heels greater than one inch! I am not your average stiletto woman :)

The physio was also a little concerned about the fact my right calf was much colder than the left (despite I suppose much use of ice over the last 24 hours). I was instructed to return to A&E if this leg became any colder, or swelled up.

I was then issued with an appointment for 'remedial physio' at my local leisure centre where they have physiotherapists from this hospital.

This physio also reiterated she thought it would be at least 4–6 weeks before I was dancing again. Walking at this point seemed a luxury.

I felt very low later on in the day when I thought of my Monday ballet class and missing my place in that studio and the friends I have there.

I elevated my leg and switched on the TV, preparing to exercise the remote control. (Isobel Knight)

I remember just how isolated and lonely I felt after that injury and the sense of loss. Injury has been described at times to being akin to bereavement, and yet this seems almost irrational in a non-professional dancer. What 'right' did I have to feel this sense of devastation that I truly felt after this calf tear? I suppose that I had worked very hard to get to even that point and that this was a major and unplanned blow and not part of my plans to be a fit and toned classical ballet dancer once again.

'The only way to truly overcome an injury is through a process similar to the one I went through – a thorough re-examination of one's own organisation' (Newell 1999, p.9). This is exactly what I had to do following my own injury. During the first week that it happened I decided then and there to apply to do an MSc in Dance Science at Trinity Laban. I had visited Trinity Laban once in 2006 and met both the MSc programme leader and also the senior physiotherapist while they were conducting end-of-year screening assessments with dancers. I was then struck with just how impressive Trinity Laban was, not least because of its award-winning building, but the dance science laboratory seemed amazingly ahead of its time and I knew back then I wanted to come to Trinity Laban. So here I was in 2008 applying to do a course which I hoped might just answer why I was regularly dancing in a great deal of pain and experiencing both minor and major injuries.

My initial recovery in terms of the calf was partly physio related, but initially mainly owing to Bowen therapy (see Figure 10.4), and I admit I have a bias in this, because I am a Bowen therapist, but the box opposite outlines what my blog says.

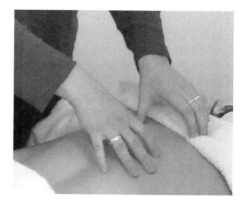

Figure 10.4: A Bowen 'move' on the upper back

Ever since the injury I had been giving myself daily sessions of the Bowen technique for my injury. It is normally against protocol to re-treat the body within 5 days of a treatment unless there is a re-injury, but since extreme heat or cold are supposed to negate Bowen, I decided that the daily reapplication of ice was in itself a good reason to continue to treat myself daily. I also believe that this was improving the speed at which the calf was healing itself which was confirmed by the physiotherapist who couldn't believe how well I was walking when he saw me ten days after the injury.

I saw the remedial physiotherapist for the first time today – 20th February. It has been ten days since the calf tear. I gave him the crutches back and said, 'I no longer need those!' and he said, 'So I can see!' I explained what I had been doing to self-treat and he was clearly impressed with how quickly the calf had been healing. He made various assessments and checked my range of movement and that there had been no trauma to the Achilles tendon, which there hadn't. He then proceeded to do some very painful deep-tissue massage on the spot of the tear to ensure no scar tissue was laid down. He couldn't do much of this because I was yelling too much and later did more Bowen to myself.

Where this physiotherapist came into his own was in giving me some remedial exercises. I requested exercises and was given some calf stretches to bulk the muscles to the injured right leg. Apparently the muscle bulk was much greater to the left than the right, which I had never noticed, or even felt upon palpation myself.

I was given two different sets of exercises one lowering the right leg on its own slowly from a rise to do six times, hanging off some stairs, and then to start with 4 rises from a bent leg, again hanging off some stairs, to give a good stretch to the soleous muscle.

I was then given the magic news that I had recovered so well I could start dancing again the following Monday if I was very careful and did no allegro or demi-pointe work. The physio trusted I knew enough about the body etc and healing to take great care. Having been originally told I wouldn't be dancing for 4–6 weeks and be back after 2, this was very good news indeed! (Isobel Knight)

Unfortunately my happiness in returning to class so soon was quite short-lived. For some strange reason, and despite my bodywork knowledge (which appeared to go out of the window), I just couldn't understand why indeed I was unable to dance as I had two weeks before tearing my calf muscle. The fact that the tissue would still be healing and therefore rather fragile, that my body would be compensating for the injury, seemed an enigma to me. My blog documents this clearly.

On 12th March I had my physio review; three weeks after the initial remedial exercises were given. The physiotherapist was impressed by how well I was managing and that the calf had healed. He said that given the sensitivity of the other calf, that any future injury risk was now as great for the left leg as for the right leg. He also said that the right leg muscle was 'bulking up nicely'. He discharged me, suggesting that I continued with the calf exercises and to contact him if there were any further problems. He said I could also start jumping again and demi-pointe work, as I felt comfortable.

After I had been back to class for a few weeks, I started to become impatient and frustrated about the fact I still couldn't do demi-pointe work or allegro very easily, and that I still couldn't completely 'trust' my leg. I began to wonder when I would get my body back to its pre-injury state.

In early April, my left calf decided to issue me a 'red card' and give me an ultimatum. It said that, 'It is unfair of you to expect me to cope with this work load and I just want you to stop and think about it. I am going to make myself as sore as possible so you are completely inhibited today!' It did that and left me to it.

Seriously though, it was a beginners' ballet class on Monday 7 April, and I was not doing any allegro or demi-pointe work again and now this was the 'good' leg having a grumble.

I felt disconnected all class long and miserable that I couldn't dance 'properly'. I was also worried about this flaring up again having historically suffered from recurrent calf-pain as a teenager.

I decided that enough was enough and made an appointment to see a specialist dance physiotherapist, which I did the following Monday. (Isobel Knight)

USE OF PHYSICAL REHABILITATION (PHYSIOTHERAPY) FOR HMS

I was accepted at Laban to start the Msc in Dance Science, but my attendance at Trinity Laban started sooner than the 2008–2009 academic year: it began with physiotherapy with senior physiotherapist Katherine Watkins in April 2008. From a recent interview with Katherine, I reflected with her how I had thought that I would have five or six physiotherapy sessions and be back to 'normal' dancing, including allegro. Katherine explained why this was so unlikely. She realised that in my case the calf wouldn't get better until she treated the supporting system. The first six months of treatment was deemed to be rehabilitative or facilitative physiotherapy, and I was given lots of exercises to do to provide some global stability, so there were many exercises for hamstrings, gluteals, adductors and abdominals. At this point, Katherine said, 'Your muscular physique changed fairly quickly, but I couldn't do hands on at that stage, because it made the tissues too irritable and painful.' In terms of a treatment plan, she suggested that fundamentally it was 'core stability, core control, control of my vast range of movement and proprioceptive control' (Katherine Watkins, personal communication, 22 April 2010). Here are some extracts from my blog over that first few months of treatment.

The exercises I was given on 12 May have been hard work. Very hard work actually, and have taken considerable dedication and time from me. I think that there will be a payback though. I suppose the first payback is in not having any injuries this month. I am also starting to feel considerably stronger and more stable on the right leg, which feels really good; particularly in the centre.

Tuesday, 9 September 2008

Here is where I am at and what I am still doing usually 6 days a week.

- Hip Flexor exercise – 4 x extensions on each leg (from lying supine)
- Oblique curls – 100 each session

- The Clam – 4 with left leg, 8 with right hip/leg
- Adductor exercise – 25 reps with each leg for those killer inner thighs!
- Hamstring exercise – 40 on right leg on its own first, then both legs slow speed, and bringing legs up to bum, fast speed
- Gluteal exercise – 10 reps on left side, 22 on the right side
- Calf exercise – 20 reps on right leg only, 4 reps on each leg for Achilles stretch
- Squats – no set number, just until my legs are tired
- Side stretches – 5 on both sides, approx 3 x a week
- Transfer of weight in turn-out – to right only and not as many times a week as it should be – 5 reps each time.

(Isobel Knight)

At some points I was spending 30–40 minutes per day doing physiotherapy exercises during the summer and autumn of 2008.

Yet I needed to do this to gain even a small amount of control in my body. Reflecting back now, my calves and quadriceps were my only functioning muscle groups. I had weak gluteals, adductors, hamstrings and abdominals. I 'screwed' my turn-out and was taking it all below the knee because nothing above the knee was functioning at all. It is a miracle that I had not injured myself more significantly in the past – although I was suffering minor tear after minor tear to my calf and was certainly injuring them in my teenage years.

By the autumn of 2008 I was certainly making some experiential connections to how my body felt and being hypermobile, but at that point I still didn't know I had HMS. My blog says: 'I wish I could stand properly without going into my hyperextension, but it is physically impossible, even if I pull up my quads. It is all too awkward!'

I also started doing Pilates in a studio as opposed to just mat work which I had done in the past. I was very fortunate in two ways. First, in the expertise of the Pilates instructors I have worked with at Trinity Laban, who are used to hypermobile students, and second, in terms of cost because I was paying student rates for this state-of-the art service which would have normally cost far more. Katherine suggested I attended initially to use the reformers to help me with my allegro (jumping steps). (My physio and Pilates story continues in Chapter 11.)

PILATES FOR HMS

Before Trinity Laban, I thought there was a right and wrong way to move and my body was always making the wrong moves. We were taught in the first five weeks about making choices and how to access these choices, and now I can make these choices and do different things and to move more effectively and efficiently. How I choose to lift my leg – makes me more efficient and having a more anatomical way to do things, and there is a more efficient way and it makes me less tired. It is not like your body was wrong or failing, which doesn't make you feel bad. You have to be really patient in Pilates and there have been times I have been in pain and the instructors are so patient. One instructor said to be calm and, don't worry, it'll come eventually. (Zinzi Minot, contemporary dance student, Trinity Laban)

I initially remember feeling that the studio sessions might be much easier than the mat-work sessions and there seemed to be so much emphasis on me feeling comfortable – I just thought that the cushions and pillows were self-indulgent. Up until now, Pilates had often been painful and gruelling work – there seemed to be no room in the past for comfort and pillows until I started to realise that these were there for alignment purposes as well as comfort. I also felt that being on a machine was 'taking the easy option' and I didn't initially understand they had a distinct purpose and that it was a totally different way of working. In fact the whole experience felt quite difficult for me for those first few sessions. I wasn't used to being watched like a hawk, I already felt I had done Pilates for quite some time and didn't understand why I had to do really 'basic' things again like roll-downs and pelvic tilts. I now believe I was doing what might have been classed as 'Intermediate Pilates' but I was probably doing it very externally, and not really fully understanding the purposes of the movement or internalising and 'embodying' the movement. Now, two years later, I still find the pelvic tilt a challenge to do properly.

In my case it has also taken a very long time to get into working into the deep core muscles as I was only really working the superficial muscles. Under close supervision, and lots and lots of practice and tuition, I am now working at a very different level, and as for the cushions, they are now my best friends, especially when I am doing 'The Clam', an exercise I find challenging, which works primarily on the gluteus muscles.

In terms of using 'The Reformer' for jumps, I did still work on that fairly early on but was not jumping on it or using it for that purpose as I had first imagined, but for improved biomechanical tracking and leg toning and strength. I am still working on this two years later, although I am now making significant progress in engaging my hamstrings and not hanging into my hypermobile or 'swayback' knees as I was in the past. The problem now is in bringing in all that I learn and experience in the Pilates studio into real life and ultimately the ballet studio. When Katherine has given me new physiotherapy exercises, it seems to take about three months before I utilise that new-found strength and probably a further three months before it gets anywhere near the ballet studio. This is all anecdotal, and I couldn't prove it.

Aside from the benefits of improved muscular strength, Pilates has been instrumental in improving my proprioception (see Chapter 2 for an initial explanation about proprioception).

PROPRIOCEPTION

When a dancer is injured, the entire body is affected, including the proprioceptive system. By rehabilitating this system as a part of a comprehensive rehabilitation plan, the chance of re-injury or chronic dysfunction is reduced. (Russell 1992, p.37)

HMS dancers had the following comments to make with respect to their proprioception.

It is terrible. Dreadful! So bad! I don't just know what is happening. I don't know where legs are when they are behind me and I have now developed a horrible habit of sickling my feet because I turn to look at them and now I have to fix that. I feel like to the front my legs are extended, but it is so hard to the back. (Zinzi Minot, contemporary dance student, Trinity Laban)

It is not great, but compared to non-dancers, my proprioception is good. It has taken me a while to 'get it'. Doing closed-chain exercises in Pilates has helped and sensing things with eyes closed. (Mari Frogner, contemporary dance student, Trinity Laban)

A somatic practices and dance movement therapist writes: 'Proprioceptive training is a form of re-education in which complex movement patterns are broken down into simpler components that are practiced, and then an attempt is made to rebuild the complex total movement pattern' (Batson 1996, p.7). This is absolutely critical in HMS patients and dancers where the sense of self and proprioception is impaired.

A Pilates instructor at Trinity Laban describes in the following how Pilates work can facilitate proprioception.

Sometimes I can put someone in a space where they haven't been before and I can see the fear in their eyes because the system is actually disorientated. And it needs to be done gradually so people can actually adapt to their new being because you are shaping a new organisation every moment in time and that reorganisation of the neurological feedback is very important and needs to be done gradually. (Mary, personal communication, 25 May 2010)

Since I have been having physiotherapy and Pilates and being taught by ballet teachers who are aware of the challenges in teaching hypermobile dancers, my proprioception is finally beginning to improve. Regular practice is also needed in making this connection (see Figures 10.5 and 10.6) and strength work is also critical. Dance students attending knee-strengthening classes for those with hypermobile knees showed an improvement and fewer injuries if the hypermobility was better managed (Sharp 2008).

Thursday, 30 July 2009

I am experiencing two separate problems. One is that in not using the mirror, I no longer have visual feedback on what the back of my right leg and my right hip (line) are doing, so had no idea, for example, that on Monday I had been going into extreme hypermobility on the right-side, and I had no idea how to pull myself out of it, or I couldn't understand how to correct what T wanted me to do.

On Tuesday, T had corrected my shoulder line, but then came around to me several times when the right leg was my supporting leg and applied finger pressure to my hamstrings and lower gluteus rotating muscles, which were apparently totally inactive. I had peered down my leg to look and she told me that she wanted me to 'feel' the difference. The trouble is that I am getting so little sensory feedback from my right hamstrings, especially at the top of the leg; I cannot yet make the connection in class. When T activated the points it definitely helped, but the muscles fatigued off very quickly, and I was in some pain later on in the class. (Isobel Knight)

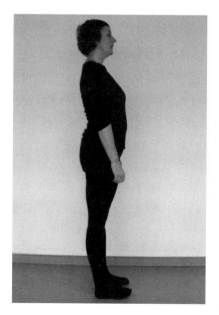

Figure 10.5: Into extreme hyperextension

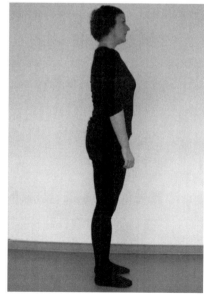

Figure 10.6: Hyperextension corrected

Use of mirror

'I specifically don't want you to look in the mirror,' says a teacher. 'You have got to be able to understand your shape from inside yourself.' (Jessel 1979, p.49)

Since proprioception is about having a sense of one's self in space, the mirror which is so commonly found in dance studios can potentially be a double-edged sword in terms of being a help and a hindrance to HMS dancers and other individuals. It might be useful to observe a very simple movement and identify an error – for example, raised hips – but in terms of going into hyperextension of the knees, sensory feedback might be more effective than visual confirmation.

For some reason, I am fascinated by observing my body in the mirror, very definitely not my face, but my body, and I think it is because I lack an internal sense of where I am, so I look for an external verification of what is true. I also have no sense of the height of my legs, so I perceive I have my leg at 45 degrees, but is far more likely to be at 90 degrees. Again, this all links back to impaired proprioception (see Figure 10.7). However, most dancers have a habit of looking in the mirror, for good or bad!

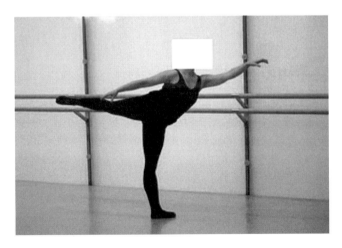

Figure 10.7: Dancer in arabesque

HANDS-ON CORRECTION AND USE OF TOUCH

In terms of my own work on proprioception in ballet, I find it incredibly challenging because there are parts of my body that are hyposensitive and, even when I am given hands-on correction, I can't always sense what is going on and promptly forget it afterwards. A discussion with Teresa Kelsey (13 May 2010) revealed this is a common problem. She says, 'Hypermobile dancers can respond there and then through touch, but they have difficulty in maintaining a correction. They seem to find it hard to retain the correction once the teacher has walked away.' Perhaps the reason why dancers find it difficult to retain correction again relates to poor proprioception. However, other hypermobile dancers also find the use of touch and hands-on corrections invaluable.

> I find hands-on corrections very helpful and respond a lot to touch to reinforce placement, and in moving me to the correct place is very effective. (Mari Frogner, contemporary dance student, Trinity Laban)
>
> Touch – that does really help. I know that my body understands corrections quite fast. I know if someone says 'drop your hip' I can do it. (Zinzi Minot, contemporary dance student, Trinity Laban)

USE OF TAPE

I have only been 'taped up' on a few occasions and it has been taping to my lumbar spine to provide it with some support and to stop me hinging in it. I loved the tape, but it is not a long-term solution because muscles should ideally be supporting the area. Taping can also help with proprioception; for example, in dancers with the swayback knee it is recommended that they should be:

> taping an 'X' behind the knee joint when it is ever so slightly flexed. Then, when the knee is hyper-extended, the tape pulls on the skin, giving immediate sensory feedback regarding the misalignment. (Fitt 1996, p.249)

Anecdotally one physiotherapist at a leading ballet school has told me how she has also taped students' thumbs and how after a few days they do start to get the idea of where the joint should be held in an attempt to help with sensory proprioception.

In her workshop on Hands Free – 'articulate the arms, wrists and fingers for magnificent presence and injury-free dance' at the 2010 International Association for Dance Medicine and Science (IADMS) conference – Stacey suggested the use of red stickers placed in the forearms of dancers when weight-bearing on arms, for example in weight stabilisation work. Stacey says that the red stickers should always be 'kissing' or facing each other – this strategy would be advantageous to hypermobile contemporary dancers who hang into their hypermobile elbows (see Figure 10.8).

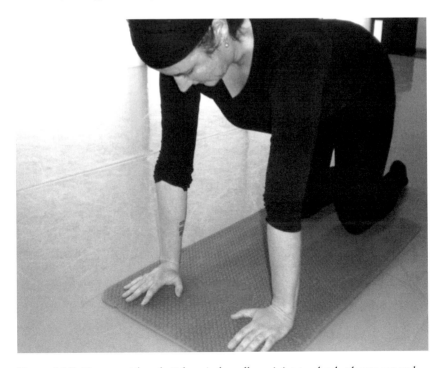

Figure 10.8: Dancer with red stickers in her elbow joint to check placement and stop going into her elbow hyperextension

IMAGERY

Although I have not yet found any imagery for my legs behind, one ballet teacher suggests the heaven and hell connection, hell with your feet, and reaching to heaven with your head, and I have found that helpful. (Zinzi Minot, contemporary dance student, Trinity Laban)

The use of imagery is very important in dance and an effective image could be really beneficial in managing some aspects of hypermobility with reference to alignment and proprioception. In the past I have had some ballet teachers suggesting to me to imagine that there are pockets of air behind my knee joint in an attempt to prevent me going into my hyperextensions of the knee. Hamstring, gluteus and adductor engagement is also critical, but this is very difficult when one has no sensory feedback, so this is another reason why imagery might be helpful:

Ideokinesis (imaging) is especially effective in controlling hypermobility when the dancer visualizes a line of movement that serves as a mechanical axis for the movement goal. (Batson 1992, p.54)

A dancer and movement educator, Eric Franklin, has written several extremely useful books about the use of imagery and dance. However, there is no reason why the use of imagery could not also be used for non-dance HMS patients in terms of describing movement. Some Pilates instructors will use imagery and even physiotherapists:

When doing exercises under instruction we are apt to think that we move or direct the moving of the muscles. What actually happens is that we get a picture from the teacher's words or his movements, and the appropriate action takes place within our own bodies to reproduce this picture. The result is successful proportion to our power of interpretation and amount of experience, but more of all perhaps to the desire to do. (Franklin 1996, p.36)

Imagery can also be used as a way of rehearsing movement without necessarily performing it. The brain is an amazing tool in this capacity and it is therefore a very good way of conserving energy and mentally imaging movement. Imagery would also be useful in terms of facilitating spatial awareness and balance for HMS patients and dancers and might help with things such as the use of first position.

Use of first position and ronds de jambe à terre

The use of first position can be particularly difficult for some HMS dancers with hypermobile knees and there has been debate about whether hypermobile dancers should leave a small gap in the heels to allow for some sensation and more effective usage and engagement of the adductor muscles (see Figures 10.9 and 10.10) and to close the gap over time as the dancer is better able to engage the adductor muscles and hamstrings, which are frequently weak in hypermobile dancers (Lawson 1973; McCormack 2010).

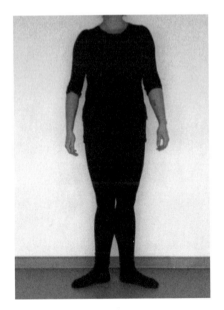
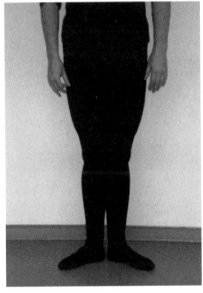

Figure 10.9: Usage of the first position with a (large) gap

Figure 10.10: The same dancer corrected with use of adductors

Exercises in classical ballet that require the dancer to go through the first position can also be a resultant challenge, but this will also depend upon the leg shape, the degree of knee hyperextension and how well the dancer manages the control of the range of movement (Figures 10.11, 10.12 and 10.13). Re-education is certainly possible, but takes patience, time and the support and guidance of an experienced teacher (McCormack 2010).

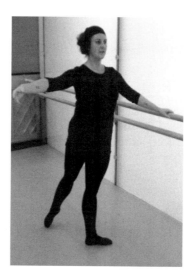

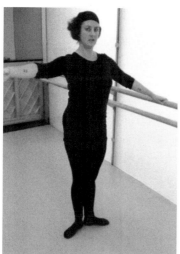
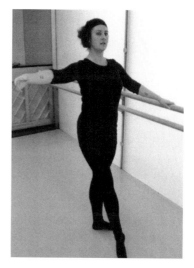

Figures 10.11, 10.12 and 10.13: Dancer doing *ronds de jambe* – note the 'corrected' first position. Red squares are in the elbow joints to also remind the dancer to soften the elbows!

BALANCE

Working out the balance is hard and working out which muscles can hold it. It is hard to find the halfway point. (Mari Frogner, contemporary dance student, Trinity Laban)

The 'halfway point' is what is so difficult for hypermobile people. The line between a neutral aligned balance and going into the extremities of the hyperextension is a fine line, but so difficult to achieve in actuality and linked to poor proprioception and insufficient muscular strength. I loathe standing in retire on the *demi-pointe* (see Figure 10.14) because essentially my plumb line feels wrong because of my knee alignment, yet relaxing the knees makes me feel even more insecure and out of control. I know that this is biomechanically correct, but it is a great challenge to achieve in actuality:

> When rising to demi-pointe dancers with swayback knees must hold their weight upwards and centred over the balls of the feet and rise no higher than demi-pointe…because they show a tendency to roll outwards at the ankle and thus place too much weight on the little toe and not over the three bigger toes. (Lawson 1973, p.26)

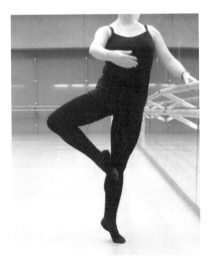

Figure 10.14: Dancer in retire

183

In terms of assessing the hypermobile dancer's ability in dynamic balance (balance in movement), a study looked at dancers performing the modified Star Execution Balance Test (mSEBT), which involves moving around a star shape (stuck on the floor); HMS dancers were slower in timed performance compared to generalised hypermobile dancers or controls. However, neither HMS nor generalised hypermobile (asymptomatic) dancers were related to SEBT reach, distance or balance error scores compared to controls. It might be that HMS and generalised hypermobile dancers have developed strategies to balance dynamically. The study recommends observing HMS and generalised hypermobile dancers' postural habits as to whether these contribute to potential injury risks (Peoples 2009). This links into observations of hypermobile dancers going into prolonged stretches and fidgeting behaviour. Unfortunately, owing to my injured calves, I never got to try the SEBT, but I suspect I would have found it quite a challenge and been rather slow at performing it – which might just relate to the increased time to reorganise my body, and less refined control, but this can only be conjecture.

STRETCHING

There is sometimes a misunderstanding about the use of stretching and hypermobility. Some dance teachers wonder why hypermobile people should need to improve upon their flexibility, and yet one of the problems for hypermobile people and dancers is that they frequently feel stiff and stretching relieves the stiffness (Simmonds and Keer 2007). Dance teachers find this hard to accept because they already perceive a large ROM and find it inconceivable that hypermobile people need to increase their extensions. It is certainly recommended that HMS dancers avoid going into 'end of range' stretches and avoid hanging into their most hypermobile joints. However, it would be futile to reprehend them for stretching and indeed it follows that, where there are areas of hypermobility, there are equally areas of hypomobility and some tight areas need careful stretching and release (Howse and McCormack 2009; McCormack 2010). Again, Pilates would be highly desirable for facilitating stretching as well as strengthening as part of the rehabilitative programme for HMS dancers and other people. A general rule of thumb that I have heard before from leading experts in hypermobility is that strength should ideally match flexibility or flexibility should (ideally) match strength.

MUSICALITY AND MEMORY

Anecdotal observations suggest that hypermobile dancers seem to have more difficulty in processing and remembering dance sequences. Since I am an HMS dancer who has been observed behaving in this manner, and following my own personal experience and research, I can only conclude that the reasons for the behaviour are that so much extra brain functioning is used to control the body that it is almost an overload to cope with any additional information. I believe that I also sometimes run very fractionally behind the music because it just takes a few crucial additional seconds to gather my body and all its extra range of movement. I have observed other hypermobile dancers running behind the music and so the reasons underlying it should be further investigated, but the most likely explanation is probably related to the delay in bodily reorganisation. I also find that anxiety is a personal issue and may also be inhibiting my memory in terms of recalling dance sequences. The more anxious I become about a sequence, the more likely I am to make mistakes. Additionally if I am particularly compensating for injury or pain (regularly) this increases the likelihood of memory and processing errors. There is certainly mounting academic research that links HMS and anxiety and the circumstantial evidence about DCD and HMS would indicate that it is not unreasonable to suggest that memory recall and processing might also be affected in the person with HMS. Indeed, other dancers that were interviewed have also reported difficulty with memory recall.

My memory is not good enough. Will remember to a point and then can't get past that point... My concentration is not very good. I drift off, even if I don't want to. All the time. I go somewhere. I don't know what distracts me. I am not thinking about something present or relevant. It always happens in ballet! I can be looking at the exercise, and think I am listening to it, then realise I am being counted in and I don't know what I am doing! (Zinzi Minot, contemporary dance student, Trinity Laban)

I have problems with changing directions and any turns, and find turns hard and changing directions and reorganising my body again. Not sure it is to do with being hypermobile, but I am very anxious about turns. (Mari Frogner, contemporary dance student, Trinity Laban)

I need to learn slowly and have been really bad at picking up movement fast. I was always one of the last to pick things up. I always felt a failure. I couldn't pick up movement sequences fast. It takes me longer than others… In terms of memory and learning, very distracted, find it hard to memorise things. I like to be slow with my body. I like slowness. It is all to do with feeling safe and being centred, then I can pick things up, and concentrate better. The fidgety distracted qualities are very present in my life. [We] hypermobile people are basically out of our centre all of the time, which is why Pilates and meditation are so important for me. Organisation of where the body is in space, coordination, neurological re-education is so important for hypermobile people and is an ongoing process. (Mary, Pilates instructor)

INJURY AND RED FLAGS

It can be argued that [hypermobile physiques] make the most interesting and stunning dancers if they are well understood, trained well at their own pace and prevented from injury. (Howse and McCormack 2009, p.69)

As already mentioned, once dancers with HMS are injured, the likelihood of future injury is predictable. The crucial aspect in an ideal world lies in preventing injury in the first place, and certainly in recognising that healing in HMS dancers takes longer and so they are more likely to endure time-loss injuries. This is why HMS dancers are less likely to make it to the top of their chosen career path. The remedial care of the HMS dancer must take a multidisciplinary approach and will need the expertise of the dance teacher, physiotherapist and Pilates team. Those who are generalised hypermobile (asymptomatic) would also be prudent to accept the same advice, although the research shows that their chances of success are higher compared to those with HMS (Briggs *et al.* 2009; McCormack *et al.* 2004; Ruemper 2008).

In terms of myself as an HMS dancer, I would like to suggest the following red flags:

- Lapses in concentration.

- Inability to follow sequences.

- Making continual mistakes or inaccuracies – even with steps I am familiar with.

- Lack of stability and balance.

- Not able to stand still, continuing to go into stretches or forward bends.

- Feeling very anxious.

- Feeling fatigued.

- Being injured already and compensating for an injured body part (distraction).

- Menstrual cycle influence (progesterone increases joint laxity).

Further research would need to prove how many of those themes were common among other HMS dancers and patients, but if we could start to predict injury we could also become better at preventing it through strategies such as imagery, Pilates, interceptive remedial physiotherapy and even psychologically.

CONVEYING MESSAGES TO DANCE AND PILATES TEACHERS

There are times when I have been occasionally ridiculed having explained to ballet teachers, Pilates instructors and medics that I cannot do something. It is in my personality to 'try' and certainly to work hard. I therefore find it upsetting that someone would think that I am making any less effort and tell me 'I could do more' in a physical sense than I am already doing at that moment. For example, I was doing an exercise for strengthening the spinal muscles (on standing) and I was asked to push the teacher's arms away. I was using all possible muscle power at the time, and the teacher said to me, 'Come on Isobel, you can do more than that.' When I showed the exercise to Katherine (my physiotherapist) she said that there was no way I could do more; there was nothing to push against because I was already completely unstable in that area! I am not sure how better I could have responded to that teacher, and why she didn't understand that I was working maximally. Teachers, instructors and some medical professionals do need to understand that in general the hypermobile person will be trying really, really hard – it is just that there is very often limited power owing to the tissue laxity and weakened muscles. Psychologically being told you should be doing more when you physically cannot is quite difficult and sometimes upsetting.

Dance teachers and Pilates instructors may need reminding that the HMS dancer will have far greater difficulty with endurance owing to weaker core and stabilising muscles and slow-twitch (endurance) muscles (Simmonds and Keer 2007). Hypermobile individuals are less able to tolerate repetition because the muscles are working harder to control an extra range of movement, which might explain why their muscles fatigue sooner than in non-hypermobiles, and they feel tired (Bird 2007b; Keer *et al.* 2003). The HMS dancer is slower to heal and is likely to miss more class time, thus putting them further behind their peers (Briggs *et al.* 2009), which (teachers are reminded) will also have psychological implications.

PSYCHOLOGY AND INJURY

The psychological implications of injury in dancers have only recently begun to receive adequate attention within the research field of dance science and medicine. In terms of hypermobile dancers there is frequently literature about improving strength and proprioception and preventing the dancer going into the extremities of their joint hypermobility (Briggs *et al.* 2009; Desfor 2003; McCormack *et al.* 2004), but the psychological implications of the hypermobile dancer who is frequently injured or missing class or falling behind other dancers in class is rarely discussed. An article on dance injury rehabilitation mentions the psychological element of injury. In injured ballet dancers, the injury types were fractures, and overuse injuries were linked to the personality type of overachiever (Liederbach 2000, p.56). This is interesting and another link with perfectionism has been found in terms of HMS adolescent dancers scoring higher in perfectionism than non-HMS dancers (Knight 2009a).

Dance psychology research suggests that certain psychological states including anxiety and perfectionism might indicate the dancer is not coping and increase the likelihood of injury, which might not be surprising in a population that has such difficult external control of their physical body (Hamilton, Solomon and Solomon 2006; Keer 2003; Simmonds and Keer 2007). It might be useful to look at potential ways for HMS dancers to manage perfectionism perhaps through use of dance psychology skills in dance training, for example the use of imagery and self-talk, or CBT (see Chapter 6), as ways of managing perfectionism (Noh and Morris 2004). In the clinical HMS population, clinicians might like to consider research into perfectionism with HMS patients so that, if HMS patients do show greater degrees of perfectionism, they can be given additional psychological clinical support.

As we have seen, there is increasing evidence to suggest links with anxiety and HMS (see Chapter 9), but there is not currently any evidence to suggest that HMS dancers suffer greater anxiety than non-HMS dancers. A preliminary study did not find any significant differences in anxiety scores of HMS and non-HMS adolescent dancers (Knight 2009a), but further research is needed to investigate the psychological impact of frequent injuries and injury rehabilitation in the HMS cohort and maximise ways of supporting injured HMS individuals.

In the non-HMS population and general 'injured dancer' population, psychological rehabilitation strategies might include imagery, self-talk (goal-setting) and perhaps in observing class, although this can sometimes be depressing for the injured dancer. The dance–practitioner relationship is crucial in injury rehabilitation and for trust in the practitioner providing the medical support (Lai and Ruanne 2008; Mainwaring, Krasnow and Kerr 2001). I can certainly concur with that from my own experience of regular injury at the helm of HMS. Chapter 9 goes into more detail about the psychological implications of HMS.

CONCLUSION

This chapter has discussed HMS and dance including practical ways forward:

- characteristics of hypermobile dancers

- what is good about being a hypermobile dancer

- difficulties for hypermobile dancers
- my experiences of returning to classical ballet and injury
- use of physical rehabilitation (physiotherapy) for HMS
- Pilates for HMS
- proprioception
- hands-on correction and use of touch
- use of tape
- imagery
- balance
- stretching
- musicality and memory
- injury and red flags
- conveying messages to dance and Pilates teachers
- psychology and injury.

The opening quote for this chapter was by an HMS contemporary dancer who described her hypermobility to be her best friend and worst enemy. Professor Grahame has often described hypermobility as being like 'the Beauty and the Beast'. In dance this could not be truer. The aesthetical component of the hypermobile line and extension is truly beautiful. The underlying pain, fatigue and injury are truly beastly. In order to succeed as a dancer a very careful rehabilitation and ongoing maintenance programme is going to be a crucial component of success; it must be incredibly carefully managed (Howse and McCormack 2009).

CHAPTER **11**

Therapeutic Support Management and HMS

Living with HMS is very much about management, of which you are the personal director. It is an ongoing work in progress, but it requires a great deal of personal strength in managing something that is at times unmanageable, just like a difficult work colleague. Sometimes the workload becomes immense (collision of symptoms) and just occasionally one needs to be 'out of the office' and take a holiday from it and 'do nothing'. In order to cope with this it is necessary to have a support team. Let me take you through mine. I have my immediate family and close friends and then I have my own medical team, some of whom I see weekly, while others much less frequently (Figure 11.1). As I see it, the better my management structure is, the more likely I am to be able to manage my own high expectations of myself in my personal, social and work life. It has taken me a long while to get to this stage, but it is working for me. I have had to understand that the reason that I work in intensive bursts with periods of quiet is that it seems to mimic my condition. I hope over time to even out the intensity with fewer peaks and troughs. This is just another form of pacing, and one of my goals in physiotherapy is to see if we can even out these extremities. I am still working towards a more even keel!

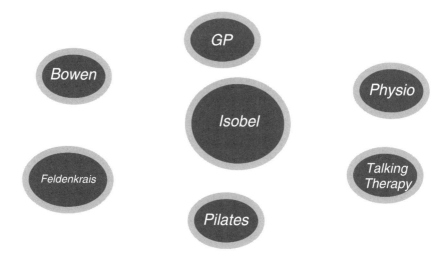

Figure 11.1: Isobel's support network

In this chapter we look at some of the forms of therapeutic support that might be helpful for HMS patients. I pick up my own journey in terms of physiotherapy and Pilates while describing and discussing a wider range of medical, complementary health and other therapeutic support available. The pacing, goal-setting and pain-management strategies outlined in Chapter 6 are all essential, coupled with the psychological information in Chapter 9, the theoretical understanding of HMS in Chapters 1 and 2, and wider-syndrome conditions found in Chapter 7. You are not alone. I mention 'Talking Therapy' in my support networks diagram, and here I am not actually implying counselling therapy, although that might indeed be useful, but just in talking to others, or perhaps in using the HMSA Forum, or talking to friends. I am meaning obtaining the support you need. You could consider your own support network and visualise what it might look like.

DIET

'You are what you eat.' In a multisystemic condition where the body is having to work very hard to constantly repair injury and 'damage' at the hands of faulty collagen proteins, the need for good nutrition and diet is crucial. Anecdotally, it seems that many of us with HMS are quicker to pick up infections and seem to have weakened immune systems. Whether this is because our bodies are always battling to repair our weakened skin and soft tissues is speculative. Perhaps our immunity also links in to impoverished sleep that many HMS patients allude to. Either way it seems that we are potentially more open to contracting infection and need to take optimal care of ourselves.

A well-balanced diet might at least increase the body's armour and defences against illness and infection and help it to respond more quickly if one succumbs to illness. It is therefore important that the diet is varied and contains adequate protein, plenty of fresh fruit and vegetables and certainly includes plenty of Vitamin C which is essential to repair and wound healing (Tinkle 2008). Adequate calcium and Vitamin D is important to promote essential bone growth and maintenance, since many of us are susceptible to bone fractures and dislocations. It is important to ensure that the diet contains all vitamins and trace minerals, many of which can be overlooked, so it might be beneficial to take a good multivitamin and mineral tablet to ensure that these are accounted for. While it is difficult to maintain a healthy weight if you become particularly inactive owing to your HMS, and I know from personal experience as I gained 20kg in weight, which I have fortunately managed to shed, there is no doubt that carrying excess weight will contribute to an increased load on an already fragile skeletal and soft-tissue system, and lead to an increase in symptoms and possibly pain as well. If you feel that your diet could be improved it might be worth seeking advice from your GP, registered dietician or a nutritionist who might also be able to advise if weight management is an issue, or to support IBS, which is known to be related to HMS (Zarate *et al.* 2009). A registered dietician might be able to support with the possibilities of food intolerances such as dairy and wheat, which are known irritants with IBS, and might advise with things such as food diaries to identify patterns and changes in symptoms. IBS can also affect back pain and related symptoms, so it is important to look at diet as part of the overall management of your HMS as a chronic medical condition.

SLEEP

Sleep – good stuff! However, so dangerous I'm surprised it's legal. I need a firm mattress, my contoured pillow, and for it to be not too hot or too cold. I also need to be locked away and left in peace. (Kay, aged 44)

Sleep – indeed! Patients with HMS do have problems. I ask people if they have a sleep problem and the majority say sleep is disturbed by pain from movement. I also ask if sleep is restorative and whether the patient wakes up feeling they have had good sleep. It is amazing how many say it isn't. This is another facet of chronic pain and sleep, and sleep is not effective in restoring the body's healing and energy. (Professor Rodney Grahame, personal communication, 20 October 2010)

Many people with HMS have difficulty in sleeping. At one level this is not surprising given that many HMS people are in pain, and pain is a terrible sleep robber. However, it is all the other things that seem to stop me personally from sleeping, such as fidgeting and restless leg syndrome, a curious phenomenon where you might feel that your limbs are itching or full of 'ants' or that the limb feels heavy and needs lots of stretching (Tinkle 2008). I regularly suffer from cramp that is sometimes excruciating to the extent that I scream. My body never seems comfortable, no matter how I lie, and although carefully positioned pillows help, including pillows between my knees, I just don't feel comfortable. An overactive bladder wakes me up to six times a night on bad nights, and so you can see why I will often watch the hour-hand of the clock pass every hour. Add in an often extremely busy head and you will wonder why I bother with lying horizontal at all. Waking up is often extremely difficult and sometimes I am so tired and sleepy in the mornings I literally don't know what I am doing and amble about my flat with my eyes shut. I am often asleep on the way to work, rather than on the way home. Caffeine is rarely the answer (not something that I cope with well in large quantities). I am often in such a chronic state of sleep deprivation that I frequently have headaches and struggle to function at all. I would say that my mental function, memory, concentration and ability to learn and process are regularly slightly impaired owing to my regular lack of sufficient sleep. Just occasionally I have some good nights including having dreams and then the world is a radically different place where anything is possible! Sadly I expect my story is very similar for many HMS patients. Sleeping pills are not really the answer, and I wouldn't mind my sleep being so difficult, but I do most of the right things in terms of getting exercise, fresh air and trying to switch off at the end of the day. I avoid caffeine after lunch and even being caffeine free hasn't improved things when I have tried that. Complementary therapy treatments have some benefits; Bowen therapy has been especially helpful in this matter and I often have a few really good nights of deep sleep following Bowen. Other therapies such as Reiki, Shiatsu and cranio-sacral therapy are also excellent in this respect.

In terms of sleep hygiene it is well known that trying to stick to a regular bedtime can help, and having a herbal tea and a warm bath before bed can help along with reading a little before going to sleep. Computer and TV should be avoided immediately before sleep. Ensuring that your bedroom is not too warm or cold is a good idea, but also free from too much mess and clutter and that mattresses and pillows are as good quality as you are able to afford – given how much time we spend in bed in a lifetime. The standard advice if you are lying down and not sleeping is that you get up and do something else in a different room. If my pain is very bad, I might go and watch part of a familiar film (not a horror) or comedy, take some painkillers, as appropriate, and then try sleeping again. One of my favourite pain-relieving strategies is to lie in the bath. It is a good job that I can't have a water meter because I regularly have two baths a day just because this is something that helps me. If I have very severe pain I might also have a third bath in the middle of the night! Other people will have their own strategies. In the end if you really cannot sleep, you sometimes have to accept that you are getting rest from lying down and that is the way I now try and view it, however irritating that is. There is no doubt why sleep deprivation is seen as a form of torture in some countries, and the effect that sleep deprivation has on mood and cognitive processing is very detrimental. The link between poor sleep and fibromyalgia and chronic fatigue is also known, which is why these conditions also seem to link with HMS. For further advice about your own sleep management, please speak to your own doctor.

PHYSIOTHERAPY

> Hypermobility does not have to be a degenerative condition, so physiotherapy can be restorative. Hypermobility is a multisystemic condition and physiotherapists need to bear this in mind and support the psychological aspect also. (Dr Jane Simmonds, personal communication, 14 August 2010)

Unfortunately my experience of physiotherapy has not always been as positive as it should have been. With the insight I now have into HMS, I believe that this is because the physiotherapists that I saw in the past just didn't know about the implications of hypermobility and certainly not about the systemic nature of HMS and how it was affecting me. Comments such as 'Your back is horrendous' are really not helpful and as a patient make you believe that you have a serious and very permanent problem. While this might be true, the way in which one hears such information impedes on interpretation and the way in which one manages such news. My back isn't really horrendous. A consultant neurosurgeon deemed it to be otherwise, despite my posterior disc bulge. Compared to the rest of the 'normal' population, my back does have an abnormal range of movement, but this feels 'normal' to me. I have excessive hinging in the lumbar spine, and my neck is also hypermobile. My thoracic spine is very tight, but logically this has to be the case just to provide me with some stability. This is very often the case with hypermobile people. It often follows there will be some areas of tightness around areas of hypermobility (Simmonds and Keer 2007). One goal of physiotherapy is therefore to gain control of the hypermobile areas, while gradually loosening and relaxing the areas of tightness in the thoracic spine, making the spine more functional, and gaining control of a large range of movement.

There are several reasons why physiotherapy is an essential aspect to managing HMS. Physiotherapist Katherine Watkins (personal communication, 22 April 2010) said that the following were the fundamental reasons behind physiotherapy and in managing HMS: 'core stability, core control, control of my vast range of movement and proprioceptive control'. In terms of range of movement, Katherine suggests that explaining 'normal' movement to me is very difficult because I have not experienced 'normal movement', so what she expects to see is not what she actually sees and she finds it difficult to communicate what she actually wants to see. Analysing quality of movement is essentially more important than quantity of movement where compensatory relative flexibility occurs as a result of 'muscle imbalances, joint stiffness, poor motor control and altered (movement) recruitment patterns' (Simmonds and Keer 2007, p.303). Excessive movement at the hypermobile segment/s can lead to instability and potentially pain and further movement and segmental imbalances. An outcome of physiotherapy can therefore be to alter incorrect movement patterns.

In terms of correcting movement patterns, this work would need to be done in conjunction with other work such as improving core stability and control. When I first started having physiotherapy with Katherine, she said that, when she first met me, she wondered how I managed to walk! I know very well that she did not mean this in an insulting or unkind way. It was just that it was almost a logical impossibility because so many of my major muscle groups such as hamstrings, gluteals and adductor muscles were not functioning. I remember that prior to 2008 my calf and quadriceps (front of thigh) muscles were holding the fort in terms of my limbs; they were often painful and sore because they were overworking at the expense of other core groups of muscles which were woefully inept at the time and almost dormant. Although by 2008 I had been doing Pilates, my abdominal muscles were still extremely weak (and are still a work in progress). It was hardly a surprise that my lower back would end up in pain when Katherine first attempted to change anything in relation to movement patterns. In fact this work was impossible for several months until I started to do some rehabilitative exercises just to get some of my stabilising muscles operational. I described in Chapter 10 some of the exercises I was given and how at some point I was doing 30–40 minutes of physio exercises a day. It is important to note that the exercises that I was given did not cause me increasing pain, although some of them were difficult to begin with until the muscles started to become acquainted with the work they needed to do. This is important since patients are more likely to comply with exercises that do not cause them increased pain levels. The exercises need to be realistic and manageable for them (Simmonds and Keer 2007). In fact, when I was doing up to 100 oblique curls per day, Katherine put a stop to me doing them because I wasn't really intending to become a body-builder!

My journey with physiotherapy has not necessarily gone about in a linear or straightforward fashion. I have at times experienced reactions to treatment, for example dizziness, or felt that I was deteriorating or not making as much progress. This is more of a perception than a factual truth, and of course my body was and still is making lots of progress; it is just that change to the body is just as overwhelming as it can be with changes in life – for example moving house or changing jobs. My body has had to go through major changes in order to make improvements to my biomechanical functioning. Owing to the holistic nature of HMS, what I thought were merely changes to my biomechanical functioning – improved hamstring strength or gluteals and postural changes – have also affected me physiologically. I have at times had vascular-type reactions to treatment, such as changes in temperature and heart rate. I believe that physiotherapy has also affected my breathing patterns and my respiratory system now functions better because my ribs move in a more functional way where they were perhaps stuck before. As my abdominal muscles work more effectively I also believe that my digestion is improving and appears less 'sluggish'. These are not things I could necessarily 'prove' – they are perceived changes. Pain management has helped me to understand why my pain is more amplified, although this is still difficult to accept – but when my pain does flare up I am better able to cope with it than I did before. The following are some extracts from the blog which has been documenting my progress through physiotherapy (and other modalities).

Thursday, 14 January 2009

I said that fatigue was an ongoing problem and also breathing difficulties – particularly in lateral breathing – I only mouth/shallow breathe at the moment. K did some more work on my neck and said that she would work around the first rib area and get into the thoracic spine – but at the moment part of that was too sore and she didn't want to do too much on me today.

Sunday, 18 January 2009

Unfortunately, and as K predicted, my back has been vile. It is very painful today, and the pain has now returned in my hip following her adjustment. I am getting to the point where I might just cope with where I have got to without all this additional pain and discomfort. Fortunately, I am a very stubborn person, and in the end my stubborn and determined streak will win through.

Sunday, 7 February 2010: physio 'al dente'

I love my physiotherapist for this. Because I had a bit of an over-reaction to my last treatment, she said that she would slightly undercook me this time and so we are now doing 'physio al dente'. K said she was using this tack with another patient, and in fact I have to do the same (now I think about it) with patients I treat with chronic fatigue and syndrome related conditions. Anyway – I like K's usual humorous approach – especially when things have been difficult lately what with vascular reactions and muscle spasms. Humour is sometimes just the very best tool there is – no wonder 'Laughter is the best medicine'. (Isobel Knight)

In addition to helping with controlling a large range of movement, movement repatterning and core control, physiotherapy also helps with proprioceptive control (Simmonds and Keer 2007). Proprioception is about understanding where we are in space (see Chapter 2) and proprioception is often impaired in HMS patients, which can feel extremely disorientating.

> Proprioceptive training is a form of re-education in which complex movement patterns are broken down into simpler components that are practiced, and then an attempt is made to rebuild the complex total movement pattern. (Batson 1996, p.7)

After I had been doing rehabilitative exercises in physiotherapy for a while and was starting to improve my core stability and control, Katherine and I started to work on my proprioceptive control.

Thursday, 15 January 2009

K said that I had all the ingredients of a recipe working separately, but not integrated in a dish yet. She said that she would like me to now be working more neurologically, rather than just muscularly – hence the proprioception work. In Pilates she wants me doing lots of wobble board work and anything that challenges my balance, and taking my limbs out of hyperextension.

Sunday, 21 June 2009

Finally, last week I managed to do some 'one-legged' balances on the wobble board without holding on! This is a major achievement since not so long ago (March) I couldn't manage to stand on the wobble board and balance with both legs. Still, I do think that it depends on the day, on my proprioception and how 'hypermobile' my legs feel!

Saturday, 21 November 2009

Both K and M are ensuring I do plenty of proprioceptive work 'without use of the mirror'. M also helped me with side bends today. The problem side is always the right! The bilateral differences are still very great. (Isobel Knight)

I originally started to have physiotherapy in order to rehabilitate my injured calf, but I cannot believe how very much longer my treatment course has taken and just how much there has been to address owing to systemic biomechanical failure at the mercy of my HMS. I have often felt a hypochondriac because of the number of different injuries that have arisen, or ones that haven't healed in the past that have reared their heads again. The acute episodes of fatigue that I have experienced while my body has been reorganising itself have at times been very difficult, as is the changeable nature of my hypermobility, which might be hormonally linked (see Chapter 8). There are some days when I find it exceptionally difficult to avoid complete collapse into my joints on my particularly 'hypermobile' days.

My physiotherapist said the following to me.

I almost expect you to return to clinic with other injuries/problems, but an interpretation of hypochondria was entirely your own view, and not my view… You (and other HMS patients) have to be mentally very, very strong. (Katherine Watkins, personal communication, 22 April 2010)

More entries from my blog follow.

Friday, 11 September 2009

It is interesting that as soon as I get too tired of a particular exercise I just go straight into my hyperextension to relieve the pain and muscle fatigue, but that is presumably because I lack endurance, as the literature suggests. Anyway, the fatigue is very real, and at times I do feel like I have been run over by a bus. It lasts a few hours/days, and then goes away. Today I am wondering 'why bother' with my muscles since it sometimes feels easier to collapse into my joints. Also I find my knees are so much stronger in their hyperextension than when they are removed from it. My knees are like wobbly jelly when they are not hyperextended. If K, T, and M read this, they will definitely tell me off. Maybe I should dance completely bandaged up!

I am so fatigued today – there are several reasons why this is, but one of them relates to standing around a lot yesterday, while at work for a press-launch. I end up fidgeting, standing with my legs crossed, leaning on one leg and sitting in at the hip. My back also aches because my abdominal muscles cannot cope with supporting me for any great length of time. I am definitely better if I move about – although I am much better in some seated positions in terms of sustaining postures, than others. I love sitting with my legs crossed on the floor, and if I have a wall to lean on, that is even better.

Monday, 2 November 2009

The trouble when one is injured is that the longer the injury remains, the more biomechanical compensations end up being made. Something that started as a sharp pain in my right hip is now creating pain in my left knee and heel and calf and my back as I make negotiations in avoiding too much weight transference onto the right hip...

...Chronic pain is classified in instances lasting for duration of more than 3 months. Interestingly you might wonder why I am not resting totally – well I did and it made the pain even worse. It seems that heads and tails I lose...

I am seeing K again and would like to know if she is able to make a better diagnosis of what is going on. I would really like to solve the problem because I am not far off from struggling to walk and yet I will still try and dance just because I want to and because I am so terrified of losing my muscle tone.

...I have spent several days learning lots more about hypermobility and exercises – but at the moment I am feeling that my need for support is more about pain management and emotional management since I am feeling on the edge of tears and can't face the fact I might have to stop dancing. Again. (Isobel Knight)

Now, after two and a half years of physiotherapy (on and off), I am starting to feel generally more in control of my body and my life. Continuing with physiotherapy will be necessary in order to manage my condition and to support my passion for ballet and so that I am able to continue with 'normal' activities. I continue to amuse Katherine with comments such as 'I feel stiff' with the vast range of movement that I have. My lower body is infinitely better organised and is biomechanically functioning much better than it did prior to 2008. My work with Katherine will continue for quite some time yet. I am still in the middle of my journey, and who knows where it will end up, but I am extremely grateful to her for not giving up on me and for being the physiotherapist who has helped me and made a massive difference to my functioning and quality of life. For me all those rehabilitative exercises have been worth every single repetition for an improved quality of life and so I can continue dancing. I know I will continue to get hit by waves of pain and fatigue, but understanding why this is happening has been invaluable. This is why this book has come about so that I can pass on hope and information on to other HMS people and the medical profession at large.

Tuesday, 27 April 2010: physio update

I had physio again today. At the moment, and while my body is in a good space and not over-reacting too much I am having physio weekly. K is actually able to follow her treatment plan and we are working on the same problem two weeks in a row, which rarely happens. My body has usually reacted in some other way, in the past. (Isobel Knight)

PILATES

In addition to physiotherapy I have been fortunate enough to have Pilates studio sessions at Trinity Laban, and (as I explained in Chapter 10) they are used to working with hypermobility per se and dancers, so ideal for me. Given the departmental link between Laban Health and Laban Pilates, the Pilates team were able to work closely with Katherine and to support and complement what I was doing in physiotherapy. The difference between Pilates and physiotherapy is that Pilates is working in a more holistic way in the session – so that exercises will target the whole body rather than in physiotherapy where I am usually getting specific exercises for certain muscle groups at a time. Eventually this is holistic, but in a Pilates session one is going to spend time doing a range of exercises, such as for the neck or feet, but all exercises stem from a similar premise of ensuring that the abdominal muscles and pelvic floor muscles are engaged in order to provide the body with core stability, something that is often very weak in people with HMS. Although many exercises might be given to strengthen weaker muscle groups, particularly stabilising muscles such as the gluteals, Pilates will also work on the stiffer and less functional areas of the body. There is then an element of stretch-related work which is just as essential for HMS and non-HMS people. Pilates works holistically and somatically and might help with improved breathing. Some people might find it very helpful in just connecting in with their body, which is the value of somatic-based work. A simplified definition of somatics might be 'bodily based access to information about the whole system and its interactive patterns, or, very simply, knowing oneself from the inside out' (Fitt 1996, p.304). Pilates might well enhance mood and wellbeing and have a 'calming' effect on the body. More research is required to provide this essential form of bodywork with the acclaim it deserves. Some of my key moments in Pilates since May 2009 are described below.

Tuesday, 5 May 2009

In Pilates M and I were quite surprised by how much weaker my right hamstring is – so much so that she had to help me in lowering my leg (leg attached to springs to lower). However after doing all this extra hamstring work my legs felt stronger and I was less inclined to go into my end range hyper-extension. I therefore think the way forward is lots and lots of hamstring work. I rarely have a sense of them engaging my hamstrings unless someone presses them (e.g. a teacher), so I get very poor sensory feedback from them. Additionally because they are tight, my pelvis is pulled down by them and my sitting posture is very poor – I don't sit on my sitting bones at all – but somewhere in my sacrum.

Sunday, 21 June 2009

In Pilates the other day, I had a further enlightenment whereby I realised (with E's help) that my leg and hip were actually two separate entities! This may seem extraordinarily obvious, but it might explain if I felt they were together why my hip flexors are so very tight. If I can image the separation, and that my leg is attached into a socket below the pelvis (as such) that I can get some length in my leg, rather than it being so 'in the hip'.

The other enlightenment I had was in realising that parts of my body could be extremely tight as well as the extreme flexibility that I am (more) used to. My left QL is very tight and we are working on this in Pilates. I think that is part of the problem with hypermobility – this extreme in some joint ranges at the expense of other inflexible and tight areas – for example my thoracic spine.

Monday, 11 January 2010

I am unwell yet again – and according to M in Pilates there seems to be some pattern with that and me going through some 'major shifts' in what is going on with my body in Pilates. If this is the case I may have to stop doing anything – because I can't keep getting ill! There is no doubt that my body has changed a great deal recently – particularly in the last 6 weeks. Firstly my hip is no longer hurting (hurrah, and touch-wood!), secondly my spine is just no longer behaving like a snake, thirdly I am now doing proper roll-downs with control and proper cat-extensions and it just seems that I am gaining some real control of my spine in general. M says I look particularly good in standing, although my lumbar spine still fatigues and collapse remains imminent when I sit – particularly as I do not sit on my bottom, but on my sacrum! In Pilates we are now doing work on hip abduction and lengthening out of my hips in all side work, so there is a waist-line gap. We are continuing to work on my thoracic spine, and all side-bends, which have really improved. M is also continuing to work on my foot proprioception and on loosening my tight calves.

Saturday, 17 July 2010

I had one of the best Pilates sessions I had had for a long time. I worked with M and we did some of the usual hamstring/pelvic tilt work but we did a very gruelling gluteal exercise which was hard work, and then a lot of reformer work and I was allowed to 'jump' on the reformer for the first time ever! Later in the session M made me stand on the reformer and bring the carriage in. This was a standing exercise for adductors. I was really nervous about doing it and thought I would lose balance and fall off, but I managed it and really proud that I did it after all. I don't think M realised how much of a big deal this was for me in terms of confidence, but it felt really good and I was doing all sorts of things without constantly going into my hyperextended knees – apart from a deep adductor stretch at the end, where I did hang into my knees! M suggested a more supported stretch, so I will have to think that through a bit more. (Isobel Knight)

FELDENKRAIS

Feldenkrais is a somatically based practice that I have personally found invaluable in helping with my movement repatterning and improved overall functioning and wellbeing. I particularly like somatic-based work because in this type of work you are given a free choice in how you work, which is rarely found elsewhere – for example, as a dancer I am told how and which exercises I am going to do, in physiotherapy I am told which exercises I should do, but in Feldenkrais, in what are called

'Awareness through movement' classes, which happen in small groups, the Feldenkrais practitioner will guide you through different movement possibilities to explore, but the way in which this is done, or not, is entirely up to the individual. According to Moshe Feldenkrais, founder of the technique:

> 'doing it well' inhibits the somatic experience because it is difficult to have one's attention on achievement and simultaneously feel what one is doing. In a Feldenkrais class there is no pressure to do well; participants have the opportunity to feel what is being done and learn about optimum efficiency. (Fitt 1996, p.329)

I very much like the fact that there is no right or wrong way, because it has often felt that my body has done the wrong things in the past. In Feldenkrais when in class we are taken through a series of movement possibilities – for example just reaching out an arm, which can be done in many ways – the movement is often repeated in a different way until the body decides which is the smoothest and most straightforward course of action. Much of the work is done lying on the floor and being covered in a blanket. It is entirely possible to just stop if one gets tired and curl up in the blanket and listen. I did a week of Feldenkrais classes centred around breathing, and one day I was extremely fatigued and the instructor very kindly suggested I stop and just rest. For me allowing myself 'just to be' was my biggest lesson that week – just doing 'nothing'.

Feldenkrais can also be done in a one-to-one capacity in what are called 'Functional integration sessions'. I had one of these during my course week and that was extremely beneficial because the Feldenkrais practitioner was able to work on things that were specific to me, but the practitioner does all the work, and as 'the patient' I could remain completely passive and inactive. I would like to recommend this amazing technique to people with HMS, because you can work within the realms of your own needs and ability and do as much or as little as you would like to do.

> Feldenkrais is extremely effective for achieving proper alignment, for preventing injuries, for recuperation from fatigue, and for relaxation, but the heart of the method is that it links mind and body by making actions more harmonious and congruent with intentions. (Fitt 1996, p.330)

The following are my thoughts and experiences of Feldenkrais.

Monday, 12 April 2010

I spent 3–10 [April] doing a Feldenkrais course. Overall I had a really lovely week helped by good company in the course group, sunny, warm weather and the beautiful beach and scenery of Cornwall. The course, which was excellent, was taught by S and focused primarily on breathing. At the start of the course we were doing some shoulder exploration work and I 'overreached' and as it turns out caused my hip flexors to grip and become very painful. It seems they were limiting me in order to protect me from over-stretching my shoulder area. My lower back also became very painful and sore for a few days while my thoracic and cervical spine area became freer, more relaxed and flexible. My lower back often becomes sore when it has to do even more work and for a few days my spine seemed all over the place. As the week went on the hip flexor and lower back pain went away and I was just left with a much more fluid spine. About 2 days into the course I suffered a few days of extreme fatigue. On the Wednesday I ended up in tears during one of the lessons but really my body was saying it couldn't do anymore and it needed lots more rest. For the remainder of that day I crashed out on the beach in the sunshine and read and slept. By the second half of the week my energy improved radically and I was left feeling very relaxed, peaceful, fluid, in no pain at all and with a wonderful range of movement in my upper spine. I had no headaches all week and felt very much better.

My one to one session of Feldenkrais was also very interesting. S said that she noticed in me and has noticed in other clients who have chronic fatigue that they overdo things in the body. She observed me doing an extra and superfluous movement in my lower rib area. Now that I am aware of this I will try and eliminate this. Since I felt so much better in the end after a week of Feldenkrais I have decided to reduce Pilates and increase Feldenkrais classes because they leave me feeling more mobile, yet much more relaxed and I do not end up feeling tight and tense and having muscle cramps.

I would certainly recommend Feldenkrais to other hypermobile patients. It involves gentle exploratory movements and exploring new and improved movement patterns. There are many rest breaks integrated in the lessons and it is possible to sleep or remain fairly inactive if one chooses to. I will keep hearing my teacher saying, 'Good, Leave it, Rest!' (Isobel Knight)

ALEXANDER TECHNIQUE

The Alexander technique, founded by Frederick Alexander, is another somatic practice which would be highly beneficial for people with HMS to try. The Alexander principle states that 'there are ways of using your body which are better than certain other ways' (Barlow 1973, p.18). The Alexander technique is about encouraging the body to work in a more efficient and economic way using less tension. It does require practice in order to change ingrained habits and so practice is required if you are serious about making changes and improvements. There is no doubt that Alexander teachers move beautifully and effortlessly and have amazing postures. Alexander technique sessions, which are one to one, usually begin with one lying on a couch and the teacher will position you 'correctly' and make gentle adjustments to each of your limbs and especially to the head and neck, which are gently raised on a soft block so that you can experience what is a correct neck and head alignment. After this you will be asked to stand in front of a chair and similar adjustments will be made with you standing, before you then begin to practise movements such as getting out of a chair. This may sound extraordinarily obvious, but the correct way to do this involves freeing the neck in order for the head to lead so that the rest of the body follows naturally. It is very hard to do this to start with and the teacher will guide you with this. It is not something that you learn straightaway, which is why people would usually have several classes. At the end of the sessions that I have taken (with different teachers) I usually feel taller, freer and calmer.

> Alexander's legacy is that enhanced sensitivity to proprioceptive input can be learned, so that the student can discriminate increasingly between efficient and injurious movement. (Batson 1996, p.7)

I believe that this is particularly pertinent to the individual with HMS, who is so easily at risk of injury owing to their joint laxity, hence Alexander sessions may be highly beneficial to try. One of my Alexander sessions in February 2009 is described below.

We went to a chair for me to practise standing and sitting and it took me a lot of courage to be moving to standing when I felt I would fall over. The idea was for me to be particularly thinking about my femur being connected to my hip bone and not cut off halfway down the leg. G also wanted me to be thinking about being off my knees and forgetting their existence. She also changed my spinal and neck posture, which felt very different to what I perceive as 'normal'.

After doing the chair work for a short while, we moved on to have me walking around the room. At first I wanted to lock into my hyperextensions when I paused in standing. G moved me out of hips and upper back so that I felt unstable. She asked me to pause on walking 'mid-stride'. I felt a ripple or wobble systemically and unstable, but not that I was going to fall as my feet were in a parallel fourth. I did this lots of times around the room, and it felt nicer as time went on, especially in my upper back and neck.
(Isobel Knight)

OCCUPATIONAL THERAPY

My only personal experiences of occupational therapy (OT) have stemmed from the support and information that I received while doing my pain management course. I am fortunate because I haven't really required things like splints, although I have been taped before. However, the occupational therapist I saw during the pain management course was invaluable in supporting my return to work and was able to advise me on a government scheme called 'Access to Work', which I contacted to provide support with the cost of taxis to and from work when I had particularly bad flare ups with pain, which at that time made public transport and a long trek up a hill too much for me, but the financial help of taxis made attending work possible. I have recently contacted Access to Work again for similar help in getting to work when I have had severe episodes of fatigue.

Occupational therapists look at very practical ways to make life a little easier where the physical (and psychological) difficulties of a medical condition can get in the way of some tasks. They can help with providing splints that might make doing tasks like cooking easier. They might also provide equipment that make tasks easier – for example pencil grips to help children with handwriting, or different cutlery to help with eating. They might also help with pacing activities and goal-setting, which was something that I needed help with (and still need reminding!) when I attended the pain management course. The following examples might highlight the immense value of OT.

When cooking I need frequent breaks because I cannot carry pans of heavy water – e.g. cooking pasta. I wear splints to help with this. (Jo, aged 27)

I got information from the website regarding wrist splints. I realised that I was contorting myself a lot at night and that obtaining a wrist splint helped to prevent this happening. (Sara, aged 34)

Seeing an occupational therapist (specialising in hand therapy) was a really positive step for managing my condition. We meet every few weeks to discuss any of my concerns and together we find ways of improving my hand function, from simple strengthening exercises to suggesting off-the-shelf or custom splints to support my joints during differing activities. More recently my OT was the first to realise I needed a corrective operation – I have confidence I'm being looked after which is very reassuring! (Nick, aged 25)

BOWEN THERAPY

The Bowen technique was founded in Australia in the 1960s by Tom Bowen, who developed his technique primarily to help his wife, who suffered from asthma. Tom also worked extensively with sports people and manual labourers as that was his background, rather than as a medical professional. He observed massage therapists and osteopaths, but the technique he developed was entirely his own and he even claimed that he had cracked the healing code of the body. Further research would need to be done, but there is no doubt that this remarkable technique is revolutionary in that it is one of the only healing modalities to cross all the meridians of the body, and encompasses many acupuncture points (Wilks 2007). Bowen moves are done across muscle and tendon fibres, and the Bowen move involves gently taking skin slack back and then applying gentle pressure (no more than eyeball pressure) to the muscle or area being worked on. The patient is asked to inhale and exhale while the therapist makes a gentle challenge on the muscle and on the patient's exhalation 'rolls' over the muscle. Another move (or two or three or four) may be made before the therapist then leaves the room and the patient briefly. The breaks are unique to Bowen technique and are an essential part of the work. The breaks are designed to allow the body to rest, for the energy generated to flow throughout the body, for the muscle stretch receptors to make a response and for the body to process the information. The therapist also leaves the room because it would seem invasive to 'watch' the patient during rest periods. Most patients are entirely happy with this when it is carefully explained to them. Children under 4 years old do not have breaks in treatment, and the parent is with them at all times. Children aged 5 to 16 may have a parent with them, but the parent is requested not to talk or interrupt the therapeutic dialogue.

Bowen is a holistic treatment and can work at all levels of the body, be it physically, emotionally or spiritually. It might well address a very wide range of health complaints from asthma to back pain, from ankle injuries to IBS (Knight 2010b; Wilks 2007). The body will prioritise the most urgent healing need, and the body continues to process information from the treatment session for up to five days following treatment. Patients are asked to return for a second treatment between five and ten days after the first treatment, with the exception of those who have reinjured themselves – I am thinking particularly of an HMS individual who might have had a dislocation. An asthmatic who has had an attack would also classify as a reinjury. Bowen is not often considered a long course of treatment, although this does vary, and people with HMS usually require more sessions because of the widespread nature of their injuries and the chronic nature of the complaint.

My experience of Bowen is that it has helped some of my acute injuries to heal more rapidly than they would perhaps have done otherwise. It has been instrumental in helping my back pain and at times been good for sleep and energy levels (see Figure 10.4 in Chapter 10). The HMS patients I have treated have suggested that Bowen is particularly good for helping with sleep, stress and anxiety, low energy levels and fatigue and also with IBS. Since Bowen is so very gentle it is less likely to injure or cause the HMS patient further pain – there are no manipulations. It can also be done through clothing as well as on to skin. Although I recognise my own biases as a Bowen therapist, I would highly recommend it for managing some of the 'related' symptoms to

HMS. I have also chosen to write about it because less is known about it compared to other complementary therapies. In an article about HMS for Bowen therapists, I have reminded them to be incredibly gentle with the HMS patient group because of our heightened sensitivity to pain and because of having more fragile skin and tissues (Knight 2010b). With Bowen less is more. A small amount of Bowen can have a very profound effect, and the more conditions and pain a person has, and the lower their energy, the less work we do. The following accounts might illustrate this.

My name is Louisa. I am 27 and at first I was hugely sceptical about trying Bowen therapy. I have been suffering with back pain for most of my life, and within the last year I have been diagnosed with osteoarthritis and disc degeneration. Several months ago in desperation from the worsening pain, I decided I would try alternative therapies as nothing conventional gave me any relief. My mother suggested Bowen therapy as she had come across it and found it to be very helpful. I thought it was worth a try although I wasn't expecting much! I have to say that after the first treatment I instantly knew something was going on. As soon as I got home after treatment the exhaustion was immense. The next day I woke up feeling more awake than I had in about a year. This pattern continued with the treatment, but each time the energy I felt in the days after treatment seemed to last longer and longer. In addition, my IBS symptoms calmed down and I felt more relaxed and less anxious. Unfortunately, my back pain did not improve; but I think that the Bowen really helped me to manage and live with my pain. Everything is easier when you have the energy and the will to stay awake! Most importantly of all, my Bowen therapist recognised my hypermobility; and rather than dismissing it as all the medical professionals had, she actually suggested it could be the cause of all my back problems. It was her advice that led me to a diagnosis of EDS hypermobility type, and after 17 years I finally have a reason why a 27-year-old can suffer from back problems that normally occur in much later life. (Louisa, aged 27)

Education of the patient is important so that they can return to activity. Return to work must be paced gradually with the appropriate support from the patient's employer and give them lots of good feedback. Shiatsu, Massage, Hydrotherapy, Reflexology can be helpful and reduce stress. Sometimes people have responded well to homeopathic support – although the evidence base is not presently strong for this. The other therapy that can be helpful is Reiki. (Dr Jane Simmonds, personal communication, 14 August 2010)

REIKI

I had a Reiki session, which was a very interesting and peaceful experience. I entered a room with a lightly scented candle and couch with a beautiful cover. I was asked to lie down and ensure I was comfortable. Owing to my 'spinal spasms' I felt it would be best if I rested my legs on some pillows to prevent any 'kick-offs'. My Reiki practitioner covered me with a blanket (at my request) and then took me through some gentle relaxation and breathing before she then used a pendulum to gauge areas where there may be some energetic imbalances. I had my eyes shut and was in a relaxed state while this was going on, and listening to some meditative music.

After a while N placed her hands under my head and left them there for some time, gradually moving her hands to be around my face, neck, chest, solar plexus area, lower abdomen, pelvis, knees and finally ankles and feet. This was all very gradual and took about 30 minutes. I straightaway felt that my head 'shut-up' when N had her hands under my head, my breathing slowed and I felt calmer. However, interestingly, when she got to the diaphragm, I felt more anxious again and my breathing and pulse-rate rose. I also had 'sensations' when N's hands were on my abdomen and pelvis, but felt much more relaxed when her hands were on my knees, ankles and feet. Although I never completely drifted off to sleep, I was certainly feeling deeply peaceful and relaxed by the time N had finished and she then told me she had finished.

Afterwards N and I discussed the session. N said that she found my head to be very calm and peaceful, and that from the knees down I was very grounded, but that all my troubles and energy were very different in the solar plexus and abdominal/pelvic area, which tallied with my various physical traumas in that area. She believes that I hold a lot of my worries in that area but had been able to move some of the trapped energy there. I talked about how unstable and insecure things had felt for me lately, what with the uncertainty surrounding my job and the stress of taking this new post on (from June). It might be that in a few days' time my physical body is catching up from the stress and trauma of the job anxieties and pain.

The session was highly enjoyable and would be an excellent complementary therapy for any HMS patient owing to the relaxation and energetic properties of the treatment. It would certainly help with anxiety and most probably pain levels. (MizzK, 9 October 2010)

HYDROTHERAPY

Both physiotherapists and rheumatologists advocate the use of hydro-therapy pools because of the supportive nature of the water.

The combination of buoyancy, support and warmth make it a very conducive arena for exercise... It can help with developing core stability and the use of webbed gloves and weights can be used to increase resistance. (Simmonds 2010, p.291)

I have been in hydrotherapy extensively in the past when I was first 'ordered' to do some exercise by a pain management specialist. I used to walk in the water a lot which sounds quite basic, but owing to the resistance of water is quite a challenge. When I tore my calf I went back to hydrotherapy again because I found I could do ballet exercises in the pool. For me this was much more specific to the type of exercise/dance I do, but difficult again because of the water resistance. Other HMS patients seem to enjoy hydrotherapy because of the warmth and support of the water.

Hydrotherapy – been massively helpful. (Bobbie, aged 21)

WHAT WOULD YOU LIKE TO SEE IN THE FUTURE IN TERMS OF RESEARCH?

I would like to think that the organisations that offer grants for research would encourage research by funding this field which is badly neglected. It is very difficult to get a grant. It would be nice to have a test we could use to diagnose the condition. This is proving more difficult than we thought – but remarkable progress in genetics in the present time and there are groups working on this. If you'd asked me a year ago, I'd like to see a centre dedicated to the condition and all aspects of it and all systems, and now that it is coming about this year at the Royal National Orthopaedic Hospital, which has applied itself to taking on some quite complex and difficult patients, this looks very promising. It has been difficult to get all the medical experts together, but they are now showing more willing. (Professor Rodney Grahame, personal communication, 20 October 2010)

I would like to see a move away from a scoring system towards looking at why people are hypermobile and the type of hypermobility – e.g. collagen structure or bony structure. My immediate thought is to concentrate research into those conditions that are associated with hypermobility and death in the twenties or thirties or in childbirth. In ten years' time we might be able to modify formation of the collagen tissues so that they are made at different speeds, e.g. in Marfan syndrome. I would also like to see improved service. (Professor Howard Bird, personal communication, 29 April 2010)

Living with HMS or EDS Type III is all about multidisciplinary and holistic management. There is no cure yet for this genetically inherited connective tissue disorder that causes such multisystemic chaos, but it is possible to manage the condition artfully and with support.

Early diagnosis would substantially help with the management and rehabilitation of the condition. I am dealing with 30 or more years of 'baggage' to go through, correct and address, which is very hard work and it takes a long time. I can manage with only small amounts of physiotherapy – either manual work or new exercises at a time. 'Less is more' and sometimes even just imaging or visualising a muscle working can be a good place to start. Even that can be mentally fatiguing!

Doing regular exercises is essential to ongoing management of the condition, but a programme would have to be individually created and carefully supervised – even with something like Pilates or Tai Chi. Exercise would help with improving strength and endurance, while also improving overall fitness and releasing positive endorphins, and for wellbeing and good health. It is also a critical pain management strategy. Exercise needs to be introduced slowly and carefully and paced up gradually (Simmonds 2010; Simmonds and Keer 2007).

The multidisciplinary nature of the condition means that the management will also be reflected in a multifaceted medical team which might comprise a rheumatologist, GP, physiotherapist and occupational therapist, or even a psychotherapist, Pilates instructor or complementary health practitioner. Patients might well require ongoing medical support from other experts such as gastroenterologists and podiatrists. The importance of good sleep and pain management cannot be overlooked or ignored.

Improvement takes time and, although I am managing significantly more now than I was three years ago, I still experience severe fatigue and pain and have days when I cannot function well at all. I am very much in the middle of my journey and so sleep, problems with muscle spasms and ANS problems such as postural orthostatic hypotension are still being investigated. The management of HMS is difficult and there is not a simple answer. Some medications might help, but it is trial and error.

The need for good support at home, school and work is essential. Continuing activities that you still enjoy and retaining hobbies are vitally important for wellbeing and creativity. Having a sense of humour is a great asset and can help in the more difficult times. I have found writing, both poetry and this book, cathartic and other people will find their own outlets for relaxation and dealing with the challenging times.

Finally, the Hypermobility Syndrome Association has an excellent and moderated online forum where it is possible to gain the support of other people with HMS online. The HMSA also has a helpline and a range of leaflets and information that the reader would be recommended to look at. Further details are in the Resources section.

References

Adib, N., Davies, R., Grahame, R., Woo, P. and Murray, K. (2005) 'Joint hypermobility syndrome in childhood: A not so benign disorder?' *Rheumatology, 44*, 6, 744–750.

ACAT (2011) 'Introducing CAT.' Available at www.acat.me.uk/ catintroduction.php, accessed on 6 June 2011.

Aziz, Q. (ND) 'Abdominal Symptoms in Joint Hypermobility Syndromes.' In *A Guide to Living with Joint Hypermobility Syndrome.* Plymouth: Hypermobility Syndrome Association.

Barlow, W. (1973) *The Alexander Principle.* London: Victor Gollancz.

Batson, G. (1992) 'Spinal hypermobility in the dancer: Implications for conditioning.' *Journal of Kinesiology and Medicine for Dance, 14*, 2, 39–57.

Batson, G. (1996) 'Conscious use of the human body in movement: The peripheral neuroanatomic basis of the Alexander Technique.' *Medical Problems of Performing Artists, 10*, 4, 3–11.

Bird, H. (2004) 'Rheumatological aspects of dance.' *Journal of Rheumatology, 31*, 1, 12–13.

Bird, H. (2005) 'Joint hypermobility in children.' *Rheumatology, 44*, 6, 703–704.

Bird, H. (2007a) 'Hormonal aspects of hypermobility.' *Hypermobility Syndrome Association*, Autumn, 1–10.

Bird, H. (2007b) 'Joint hypermobility.' *Musculoskeletal Care, 5*, 1, 4–19.

Bird, H. (2010) 'Pharmacotherapy in Joint Hypermobility Syndrome.' In A. Hakim, R. Keer and R. Grahame (eds) *Hypermobility, Fibromyalgia and Chronic Pain.* Philadelphia, PA: Elsevier, pp.19–34.

Bird, H., Walker, A. and Newton, J. (1988) 'A controlled study of joint laxity and injury in gymnasts.' *Journal of Orthopaedic Rheumatology, 1*, 139–145.

Bravo, J., Sanhueza, G. and Hakim, A. (2010) 'Neuromuscular Physiology in Joint Hypermobility.' In A. Hakim, R. Keer and R. Grahame (eds) *Hypermobility, Fibromyalgia and Chronic Pain*. Philadelphia, PA: Elsevier, pp.69–82.

Briggs, J., McCormack, M., Hakim, A. and Grahame, R. (2009) 'Injury and joint hypermobility syndrome in ballet dancers – A 5 year follow up.' *Rheumatology, 48*, 12, 1469–1470.

Bryden, L. (2010) 'The Cervical Spine and Jaw – Temporomandibular Joint – Physiotherapy Management.' In A. Hakim, R. Keer and R. Grahame (eds) *Hypermobility, Fibromyalgia and Chronic Pain*. Philadelphia, PA: Elsevier, pp.264–269.

Bulbena, A., Aguillo, A., Pailhez, G., Martin-Santos, R., Porta, M., Guitart, J. and Gago, J. (2004) 'Is joint hypermobility related to anxiety in a non-clinical population also?' *Psychosomatics, 45*, 5, 432–437.

Butler, K. (2010) 'The Hand.' In A. Hakim, R. Keer and R. Grahame (eds) *Hypermobility, Fibromyalgia and Chronic Pain*. Philadelphia, PA: Elsevier, pp.207–217.

Carter, C. and Wilkinson, J. (1964) 'Persistent joint laxity and congenital dislocation of the hip.' *Journal of Bone Joint Surgery, 46*, 40–45.

Chartrand, D. and Chatfield, S. (2005) 'A critical review of the prevalence of secondary amenorrhoea in ballet dancers.' *Journal of Dance Medicine and Science, 9*, 3–4, 74–80.

Daniel, C. (2010) 'Pain Management and Cognitive Behavioural Therapy.' In A. Hakim, R. Keer and R. Grahame (eds) *Hypermobility, Fibromyalgia and Chronic Pain*. Philadelphia, PA: Elsevier, pp.125–143.

Desfor, F. (2003) 'Assessing hypermobility in dancers.' *Journal of Dance Science and Medicine, 7*, 1, 17–22.

Dijkstra, P., Kropmans, T. and Stregenga, B. (2002) 'The association between generalized joint hypermobility and temporomandibular joint disorders: A systemic review.' *Journal of Dental Research, 81*, 3, 158–163.

Ehlers-Danlos Support Group (1997) *Types of EDS*. Revised at the Villefranche Meeting. Available at www.ehlers-danlos.org/index.php?option=com_con tent&task=view&id=4&Itemid=5, accessed on 3 May 2011.

Ercolani, M., Galvani, M., Franchini, C., Baracchini, F. and Chattat, R. (2008) 'Benign joint hypermobility syndrome: Psychological features and psychopathological symptoms in a sample pain-free at evaluation.' *Perceptual and Motor Skills, 107,* 246–256.

Ferrell, W. (2009) 'The sixth sense and joint hypermobility syndrome.' *Hypermobility Syndrome Association Newsletter,* Spring, 10.

Ferrell, W. and Ferrell, P. (2010) 'Proprioceptive Dysfunction in JHS and its Management.' In A. Hakim, R. Keer and R. Grahame (eds) *Hypermobility, Fibromyalgia and Chronic Pain.* Philadelphia, PA: Elsevier, pp.96–104.

Ferrell, W., Tennant, N., Sturrock, R., Ashton, L., Creed, G., Brydson, G. and Rafferty, D. (2004) 'Amelioration of symptoms of enhancement of proprioception in patients with joint hypermobility syndrome.' *Arthritis and Rheumatism, 50,* 10, 3323–3328.

Fitt, S. (1996) *Dance Kinesiology,* 2nd edn. New York: Schirmer.

Franklin, E. (1996) *Dynamic Alignment through Imagery.* Champaign, IL: Human Kinetics.

Friedman, P. and Eisen, G. (1980) *The Pilates Method of Physical and Mental Conditioning.* New York: Penguin.

Frusztajer, N.T., Dhuper, S., Warren, M.P., Brooks-Gunn, J. and Fox, R.P. (1990) 'Nutrition and the incidence of stress fractures in ballet dancers.' *Journal of Clinical Nutrition, 51,* 779–783.

Goodsell, D. (2000) *Collagen, Your Most Plentiful Protein.* Available at www.rcsb. org/pdb/static.do?p=education_discussion/molecule_of_the_month/pdb4_1.html, accessed on 3 July 2010.

Grahame, R. (2000) 'Brighton Diagnostic Criteria for the Benign Joint Hypermobility Syndrome (BJHS).' *Journal of Rheumatology, 27,* 1777–1779.

Grahame, R. (2003) 'Hypermobility and Hypermobility Syndrome.' In R. Keer and R. Grahame (eds) *Hypermobility Syndrome: Recognition and Management for Physiotherapists.* Philadelphia, PA: Elsevier, pp.1–15.

Grahame, R. (2007) 'The need to take a fresh look at criteria for hypermobility.' *Journal of Rheumatology, 34,* 4, 664–665.

Grahame, R. (2009a) 'Hypermobility: An important but often neglected area within rheumatology.' *Hypermobility Syndrome Association Newsletter,* Spring, 4–5.

Grahame, R. (2009b) 'Joint hypermobility syndrome pain.' *Current Pain and Headache Reports, 13*, 427–433.

Grahame, R. (2009c) 'Hypermobility is the key to performing arts medicine.' Keynote speech at the Annual Meeting of the International Association for Dance Medicine and Science, 29–31 October. The Hague, The Netherlands.

Grahame, R. (2010) 'What is the Joint Hypermobility Syndrome – JHS from Cradle to Grave.' In A. Hakim, R. Keer and R. Grahame (eds) *Hypermobility, Fibromyalgia and Chronic Pain.* Philadelphia, PA: Elsevier, pp.19–34.

Grahame, R. and Hakim, A. (2006) 'Joint hypermobility syndrome is highly prevalent in general rheumatology clinics, its occurrence and clinical presentation being gender, age and race-related.' *Annals of Rheumatic Disease, 65* (suppl. 2), 263.

Grahame, R. and Hakim, A. (2008) 'Hypermobility.' *Current Opinion in Rheumatology, 20*, 106–110.

Grahame, R. and Keer, R. (2010) 'Pregnancy and the Pelvis.' In A. Hakim, R. Keer and R. Grahame (eds) *Hypermobility, Fibromyalgia and Chronic Pain.* Philadelphia, PA: Elsevier, pp.245–255.

Gulbahar, S., Sahin, E., Baydar, M., Bircan, C., Kizil, R., Manisali, M., Akalin, E. and Pecker, O. (2006) 'Hypermobility syndrome increases the risk for low bone mass.' *Clinical Rheumatology, 25*, 4, 511–514.

Gurley-Green, S. (2001) 'Living with the hypermobility syndrome.' *Rheumatology, 40*, 5, 487–489.

Haddad, F. and Dhawan, R. (2010) 'The Knee Joint.' In A. Hakim, R. Keer and R. Grahame (eds) *Hypermobility, Fibromyalgia and Chronic Pain.* Philadelphia, PA: Elsevier, pp.224–231.

Hakim, A. and Grahame, R. (2004) 'Non-musculoskeletal symptoms in joint hypermobility syndrome: Indirect evidence of autonomic dysfunction.' *Rheumatology, 43*, 9, 1194–1195.

Hakim, A., Grahame, R., Norris, P. and Hopper, C. (2005) 'Local anaesthetic failure in joint hypermobility syndrome.' *Journal of the Royal Society of Medicine, 98*, 2, 84–85.

Hall, M., Ferrell, W., Sturrock, R., Hamblen, D. and Baxendale, R. (1995) 'The effect of the hypermobility syndrome on knee joint proprioception.' *Rheumatology, 34*, 2, 121–125.

Hamilton, L., Solomon, R. and Solomon, J. (2006) 'A proposal for standardized psychological screening of dancers.' *Journal of Dance, Science and Medicine, 10*, 1–2, 40–45.

Hamilton-Fairley, D. (2004) *Lecture Notes: Obstetrics and Gynaecology.* Oxford: Blackwell.

Harding, V. (2003) 'Joint Hypermobility and Chronic Pain: Possible Linking Mechanisms and Management Highlighted by a Cognitive-Behavioural Approach.' In R. Keer and R. Grahame (eds) *Hypermobility Syndrome: Recognition and Management for Physiotherapists.* Philadelphia, PA: Elsevier, pp.147–162.

Hardy, L., Jones, G. and Gould, D. (1996) *Understanding Psychological Preparation for Sport.* Chichester: Wiley.

Henderson, L. and Wood, R. (2000) *Explaining Endometriosis.* London: Allen & Unwin.

Howse, J. and McCormack, M. (2009) *Dance Technique and Injury Prevention,* 4th edn. London: A&C Black.

Jaffe, M., Tirosh, E., Cohen, A. and Taub, Y. (2005) 'Joint mobility and motor development.' *Archives of Disease in Childhood, 63,* 158–161.

Jessel, C. (1979) *Life at the Royal Ballet School.* London: Methuen.

Kanjwal, K., Karabin, B., Kanjwal, Y. and Grubb, B. (2009) 'Postpartum postural orthostatic tachycardia syndrome in a patient with the joint hypermobility syndrome.' *Cardiology Research and Practice,* doi:10.4061/2009/187543.

Keer, R. (2003) 'Physiotherapy Assessment of the Hypermobile Adult.' In R. Keer and R. Grahame (eds) *Hypermobility Syndrome: Recognition and Management for Physiotherapists.* Philadelphia, PA: Elsevier, pp.67–86.

Keer, R., Edwards-Fowler, A. and Mansi, E. (2003) 'Management of the Hypermobile Adult.' In R. Keer and R. Grahame (eds) *Hypermobility Syndrome: Recognition and Management for Physiotherapists.* Philadelphia, PA: Elsevier, pp.87–106.

Kinsler, E., Vande Vusse, L., Malone, M., Zacharaski, L. and Whiteside, J. (2008) 'Pelvic organ prolapse with hypermobility syndrome and operative bleeding managed with aprotinin.' *Journal of Pelvic Medicine and Surgery, 14,* 1, 65–68.

Kirby, A. and Davies, R. (2007) 'Developmental coordination disorder and joint hypermobility syndrome – Overlapping disorders? Implications for research and clinical practice.' *Child Care Health Development, 33*, 5, 513–519.

Kirby, A., Davies, R. and Bryant, A. (2005) 'Hypermobility syndrome and developmental coordination disorder: Similarities and features.' *International Journal of Therapy and Rehabilitation, 12*, 10, 431–437.

Knight, I. (2008–2010) *Dance Injury and Hypermobility.* Web blog. Available at http://danceinjuryrecovery.blogspot.com, accessed on 3 May 2011.

Knight, I. (2009a) 'A study investigating strength, anxiety and perfectionism differences between injured and non-injured dancers with joint hypermobility syndrome (JHS) and dancers without JHS.' MSc thesis. London: Laban.

Knight, I. (2009b) *The Skin Collection.* London: Chipmunka Publishing.

Knight, I. (2010a) 'Living with joint hypermobility syndrome (JHS).' *Hypermobility Syndrome Association Newsletter,* Summer, 10–12.

Knight, I. (2010b) 'Bowen for joint hypermobility syndrome.' *Bowen Hands, Journal of the Bowen Therapy Academy of Australia,* June, 26–27.

Knight, I. (2010c) 'Silent Support.' In N. Newson (ed.) *When You Hear Hoofbeats…and Other Poems.* Plymouth: Hypermobility Syndrome Association.

Knight, I. and Bird, H. (2010) 'A patient's journey – Joint hypermobility syndrome.' *British Medical Journal.* Available at www.bmj.com/content/341/bmj.c3044.full, accessed on 22 February 2010.

Lai, J. and Ruanne, Y. (2008) 'Communication between medical practitioners and dancers.' *Journal of Dance, Medicine and Science, 12*, 2, 47–53.

Larsson, L., Baum, J., Govind, S., Mudholkar, S. and Kollia, G. (1993) 'Benefits and disadvantages of hypermobility among musicians.' *New England Journal of Medicine, 329*, 1079–1082.

Lawson, J. (1973) *The Teaching of Classical Ballet.* London: A&C Black.

Liederbach, M. (2000) 'General considerations for guiding dance injury rehabilitation.' *Journal of Dance, Medicine and Science, 4*, 2, 54–65.

McCormack, M. (2010) 'Teaching the hypermobile dancer.' *IADMS Bulletin for Teachers, 2*, 1, 1–8.

McCormack, M., Briggs, J., Hakim, A. and Grahame, R. (2004) 'Joint laxity and the benign joint hypermobility syndrome in student and professional ballet dancers.' *Journal of Rheumatology, 31*, 1, 173–178.

McIntosh, L., Mallett, V., Frahm, J., Richardson, D. and Evans, I. (1995) 'Gynecologic disorders in women with Ehlers-Danlos syndrome.' *Journal of the Society for Gynaecologic Investigation, 2*, 3, 559–564.

Maillard, S. and Murray, K. (2003) 'Hypermobility Syndrome in Children.' In R. Keer and R. Grahame (eds) *Hypermobility Syndrome: Recognition and Management for Physiotherapists.* Philadelphia, PA: Elsevier, pp.33–50.

Maillard, S. and Payne, A. (2010) 'Physiotherapy and Occupational Therapy in the Hypermobile Child.' In A. Hakim, R. Keer and R. Grahame (eds) *Hypermobility, Fibromyalgia and Chronic Pain.* Philadelphia, PA: Elsevier, pp.179–196.

Mainwaring, L., Krasnow, D. and Kerr, G. (2001) 'And the dance goes on: Psychological impact of injury.' *Journal of Dance Medicine and Science, 5*, 4, 105–115.

Manore, M. and Thompson, J. (2000) *Sport Nutrition for Health and Performance.* Champaign, IL: Human Kinetics.

Martin-Santos, R., Bulbena, A. and Crippa, J. (2010) 'Anxiety Disorders, Their Relationship to Hypermobility and Their Management.' In A. Hakim, R. Keer and R. Grahame (eds) *Hypermobility, Fibromyalgia and Chronic Pain.* Philadelphia, PA: Elsevier, pp.53–60.

Martin-Santos, R., Bulbena, A., Porta, M., Gago, J., Molina, L. and Duro, J. (1998) 'Association between joint hypermobility syndrome and panic disorder.' *American Journal of Psychiatry, 155*, 11, 1578–1583.

Mears, J. (1996) *Coping with Endometriosis.* London: Shelton.

Middleditch, A. (2003) 'Management of the Hypermobile Adolescent.' In R. Keer and R. Grahame (eds) *Hypermobility Syndrome: Recognition and Management for Physiotherapists.* Philadelphia, PA: Elsevier, pp.51–66.

Middleditch, A. (2010) 'Physiotherapy and Occupational Therapy in the Hypermobile Adolescent.' In A. Hakim, R. Keer and R. Grahame (eds) *Hypermobility, Fibromyalgia and Chronic Pain.* Philadelphia, PA: Elsevier, pp.163–177.

Morgan, A., Pearson, S., Davies, S., Gooi, H. and Bird, H. (2007) 'Asthma and airways collapse in two heritable disorders of connective tissue.' *Annals of the Rheumatic Diseases, 66*, 1369–1373.

Newell, G. (1999) 'The Feldenkrais Method and the dancer.' In *Feldenkrais Im Überlick.* Germany: Thomas Kaubisch. Available at www.feldenkrais-itc. com/?p=p_13&sName=Further-Reading, accessed on 22 February 2011.

Newson, N. (ed.) (2010) *When You Hear Hoofbeats...and Other Poems.* Plymouth: Hypermobility Syndrome Association.

Nicholas, M., Molloy, A., Tonkin, L. and Beeston, L. (2005) *Manage Your Pain.* Sydney: Souvenir Press.

Nijs, J. (2005) 'Generalized joint hypermobility: An issue in fibromyalgia and chronic fatigue.' *Journal of Bodywork and Movement Therapies, 9,* 310–317.

Nijs, J., Aerts, A. and De Meirleir, K. (2006) 'Generalized joint hypermobility is more common in chronic fatigue syndrome than in healthy control subjects.' *Journal of Manipulative and Physiological Therapeutics, 29,* 1, 187–191.

Noh, Y. and Morris, T. (2004) 'Designing research-based interventions for the prevention of injury in dance.' *Medical Problems of Performing Artists, 19,* 82–89.

Norton, P., Baker, J., Sharp, H. and Warenski, J. (1995) 'Genitourinary prolapse and joint hypermobility in women.' *Obstetrics and Gynaecology, 85,* 2, 225–228.

Peoples, R. (2009) 'Comparing dynamic balance of hypermobile dance students and controls using the modified Star Excursion Balance Test (mSEBT).' MSc thesis. London: Laban.

Raff, M. and Byers, P. (1996) 'Joint hypermobility syndromes.' *Current Opinion in Rheumatology, 8,* 459–466.

Rahman, A. and Holman, A. (2010) 'Pharmacotherapy in Fibromyalgia.' In A. Hakim, R. Keer and R. Grahame (eds) *Hypermobility, Fibromyalgia and Chronic Pain.* Philadelphia, PA: Elsevier, pp.61–68.

Raj, S. (2006) 'The postural tachycardia syndrome (POTS): Pathophysiology, diagnosis and management.' *Indian Pacing and Electrophysiology Journal, 6,* 2, 84–99.

Redmond, A. (ND) *Feet – A Guide to Living with Joint Hypermobility Syndrome.* Plymouth: Hypermobility Syndrome Association.

Rothschild, B. (2000) *The Body Remembers: The Psychophysiology of Trauma and Trauma Treatment.* New York: Norton.

Roussel, N., Nijs, J., Mottram, S., Van Moorsel, A., Truijen, S. and Stassijns, G. (2009) 'Altered lumopelvic movement control but not generalized joint hypermobility is associated with increased injury in dancers: A prospective study.' *Journal of Manual Therapy*, doi:10.1016/j.math.2008.12.004.

Ruemper, A. (2008) 'The correlation between hypermobility and injury in contemporary dance students.' MSc thesis. London: Laban.

Russek, L. (1999) 'Hypermobility syndrome.' *Physical Therapy, 79*, 6, 591–599.

Russell, B. (1992) 'Proprioceptive rehabilitation in dancers' injuries.' *Journal of Kinesiology and Medicine for Dance, 14*, 2, 27–39.

Sharp, E. (2008) 'The bee's knees: Does hypermobility of the knee predispose students of musical theatre to knee injuries.' *Dance UK News, 68*, 24–25.

Simmonds, J. (2003) 'Rehabilitation, Fitness, Sport and Performance for Individuals with Joint Hypermobility.' In R. Keer and R. Grahame (eds) *Hypermobility Syndrome: Recognition and Management for Physiotherapists.* Philadelphia, PA: Elsevier, pp.107–126.

Simmonds, J. (2010) 'Principles of Rehabilitation and Considerations for Sport, Performance and Fitness.' In A. Hakim, R. Keer and R. Grahame (eds) *Hypermobility, Fibromyalgia and Chronic Pain.* Philadelphia, PA: Elsevier, pp.281–297.

Simmonds, J. and Keer, R. (2007) 'Hypermobility and the hypermobility syndrome.' *Manual Therapy, 12*, 4, 298–309.

Simmonds, J. and Keer, R. (2008) 'Hypermobility and the hypermobility syndrome, Part 2. Assessment and management of hypermobility syndrome: Illustrated via case studies.' *Manual Therapy, 13*, 2, E1–E11.

Simpson, M. (2006) 'Benign joint hypermobility syndrome: Evaluation, diagnosis and management.' *Journal of American Osteopath Association, 106*, 9, 531–536.

Spielberger, C.D. (1983) *Manual for the State-Trait Anxiety Inventory.* Palo Alto, CA: Consulting Psychologists Press.

Tinkle, B. (2008) *Issues and Management of Joint Hypermobility.* Greens Fork, IN: Left Paw Press.

Tinkle, B. (ed.) (2010) *Joint Hypermobility Handbook.* Greens Fork, IN: Left Paw Press.

Vounotrypidis, P., Efremidou, E., Zezos, P., Pitiakoudis, M., Maltezos, E., Lyratzopoulos, N. and Kouklakis, G. (2009) 'Prevalence of joint hypermobility and patterns of articular manifestations in patients with inflammatory bowel disease.' *Gastroenterology Research and Practice, Volume 2009.*

Wilks, J. (2007) *The Bowen Technique: The Inside Story.* Corton Denham, UK: CYMA Press.

Zarate, N., Farmer, A., Grahame, R., Mohammed, S., Knowles, C., Scott, S. and Aziz, Q. (2009) 'Unexplained gastrointestinal symptoms and joint hypermobility: Is connective tissue the missing link?' *Neurogastroenterology and Motility, 22,* 3, 252–e78.

Resources

ACCESS TO WORK

Jobcentre Plus
Access to Work Operational Support Unit
Nine Elms Lane
London SW95 9BH
Tel: 020 8426 3110

ALEXANDER TECHNIQUE

Society of Teachers of the Alexander Technique
First Floor, Linton House
39–51 Highgate Road
London NW5 1RS
Tel: 020 7482 5135
www.stat.org.uk

BOWEN ASSOCIATION UK

The official home of the Bowen technique in Europe.
Bowen Association UK
PO Box 4358
Dorchester
Dorset DT1 3BA
Tel: 0700 269 8324 (national rates apply)
Office open 9am–1pm, Monday–Friday
www.bowen-technique.co.uk

BOWENWORKS – ISOBEL KNIGHT

My own practice – I run clinics in South London (East Dulwich, Peckham and
Wimbledon) and Greenwich at Laban Health.
www.bowenworks.org

EHLERS-DANLOS SUPPORT GROUP

PO Box 337
Aldershot
Surrey GU12 6WZ
Tel: 01252 690940
www.ehlers-danlos.org/index.php?option=com_frontpage&Itemid=2

FELDENKRAIS GUILD

The Guild does not maintain a central postal address, but if you require a postal address, please contact:
Scott Clark
13 Camellia House, Idonia Street
London SE8 4LZ
Tel: 07000 785506
www.feldenkrais.co.uk

HYPERMOBILITY SYNDROME ASSOCIATION (HMSA)

49 Orchard Crescent
Oreston
Plymouth PL9 7NF
Tel: 0845 345 4465 (our telephone line has an answering machine 24 hours 7 days a week: we aim to reply to all messages within one working day)
www.hypermobility.org

LABAN HEALTH

Creekside
London SE8 3DZ
Tel: 020 8469 9479
www.trinitylaban.ac.uk/laban-health.aspx

Thomas Bull – Alexander technique: www.alextechnique.net
Nicky Jarrett – Reiki: http://nickyjarrett.co.uk
Isobel Knight – Bowen technique: www.bowenworks.org
Katherine Watkins – Physiotherapy: www.watkinsphysio.com
Hannah Wheeler – Feldenkrais: www.intofeldenkrais.com

LABAN PILATES

Tel: 020 8469 9482
www.trinitylaban.ac.uk/laban-health.aspx

LONDON HAND THERAPY

30 Cumberland Mansions
Seymour Place
London W1H 5TF
Tel: 07960 750888

OCCUPATIONAL HEALTH

College of Occupational Therapists
106–114 Borough High Street
Southwark
London SE1 1LB
Tel: 020 7357 6480
www.cot.co.uk/homepage

PHYSIOTHERAPY

Chartered Society of Physiotherapy
14 Bedford Row
London WC1R 4ED
Tel: 020 7306 6666
www.csp.org.uk

PILATES FOUNDATION

Pilates Foundation Administrator
PO Box 58235
London N1 5UY
Tel: 020 7033 0078
http://pilatesfoundation.com/newsite/index.php

TRINITY LABAN – DANCE SCIENCE

www.trinitylaban.ac.uk

WATKINS PHYSIOTHERAPY

Back on Track Healthcare
9 Merton Park Parade
Kingston Road
Wimbledon
London SW19 3NT
Tel: 020 8545 0965
www.watkinsphysio.com

Subject Index

Author Index